INSIDE

THE

PHYSICIAN

MIND

FINDING COMMON GROUND
WITH DOCTORS

INSIDE
THE
PHYSICIAN
MIND

FINDING COMMON GROUND
WITH DOCTORS

Joseph S. Bujak, MD

ACHE Management Series

Your board, staff, or clients may also benefit from this book's insight. For more information on quantity discounts, contact the Health Administration Press Marketing Manager at (312) 424-9470.

This publication is intended to provide accurate and authoritative information in regard to the subject matter covered. It is sold, or otherwise provided, with the understanding that the publisher is not engaged in rendering professional services. If professional advice or other expert assistance is required, the services of a competent professional should be sought.

The statements and opinions contained in this book are strictly those of the author(s) and do not represent the official positions of the American College of Healthcare Executives or of the Foundation of the American College of Healthcare Executives.

12 11 10 09 08   5 4 3 2 1

Library of Congress Cataloging-in-Publication Data here

Bujak, Joseph S.
  Inside the physician mind : finding common ground with doctors / Joseph S. Bujak.
     p. ; cm.
  Includes bibliographical references.
  ISBN-13: 978-1-56793-298-0 (alk. paper)
  ISBN-10: 1-56793-298-3 (alk. paper)
  1. Health services administration. 2. Hospital-physician relations. 3. Physicians. I. Title.
  [DNLM: 1. Leadership. 2. Physician's Role--psychology. 3. Organizational Culture. 4.
Physicians--psychology. 5. Quality Assurance, Health Care--methods. W 21 B932i 2008]
  RA971.9.B85 2008
  362.1068--dc22
                                    2008025290

The paper used in this publication meets the minimum requirements of American National Standard for Information Sciences—Permanence of Paper for Printed Library Materials, ANSI Z39.48-1984. ∞ ™

Acquisitions editor: Janet Davis; Project manager: Amanda Bove; Interior and cover designer: Scott R. Miller; Cover illustration: Michael Graham

Health Administration Press
A division of the Foundation of the
          American College of Healthcare Executives
1 North Franklin Street, Suite 1700
Chicago, IL 60606-3529
(312) 424-2800

Contents

Preface

I HAVE BEEN STUDYING and addressing issues that relate to physician and healthcare organization relationships for the past 16 years. A distillation and synthesis of my experiences and reflections is central to a course that I have been teaching for the American College of Healthcare Executives titled "Understanding and Influencing Physician Behavior: The Strategic Imperative" and central to this book. My personal journey began with clinical and laboratory research at the National Institutes of Health (NIH), followed by several years of teaching medical students and residents. I then served as the chief of the medical service at the Boise VA Hospital, where I functioned as a consulting diagnostician and specialist in infectious diseases. After spending eight years as a small-town general practitioner, I returned to the private practice of general internal medicine. I then began to progressively expand my work with Kootenai Medical Center, focusing on resource management and clinical outcomes measurement.

Over the years, I have journeyed through a number of different disciplines that have influenced my perceptions, judgments, and work. These have included continuous quality improvement, general systems theory, studies in leadership and ways of influencing behavior, observational assessments of physician culture, and complexity science and its applications to leadership and management in healthcare. As part of my work, I have studied the art of public speaking and facilitation. The breadth of my experiences and interests provides me with a unique perspective and credibility within the healthcare-provider community. I retain a part-time position as the vice president medical affairs for Kootenai Medical Center, which provides the opportunity to test my hypotheses in the real world and lends a pragmatic and practical aspect to the more theoretical and philosophical aspects of my work.

I am indebted to many people for helping to shape my views and for guiding me along the way. Many of them are mentioned at the end of the chapters. There are many others I have unintentionally failed to mention. To them I offer my apology. Each person provides a thread to the tapestry that I have woven along the way. The ideas of others have become a part of the fabric of my sense-making, and, after a while, it becomes difficult to separate their contributions from the amalgamation that has taken place.

Others have personally influenced me in unforgettable ways. Please indulge me as I mention them as a way of paying homage. Reverend George Luba, the best teacher I have ever known, is with me every time I speak publicly. Doctors Bill Miller, George Engel, and Bill Medd meaningfully shaped my medical school experience. Doctors Geoff Herzig, Mel Marcus, Larry Epstein, and Israel Stein helped make my days at the Bronx Municipal Hospital very special. Doctors Shelly Wolff, Dick Root, David Dale, and Jack Bennett were a significant presence during my years at the NIH (truly the highpoint of my academic life). I was privileged to serve as Dr. Robert Petersdorf's chief resident in medicine at the University of Washington, where Doctors Bruce Gilliland and Findlay Wallace provided wise counsel. Tom Atchison has been a friend, colleague, coach, and mentor in my attempts to grow as a public speaker and consultant. The administrative team at Kootenai Medical Center—Carmen Brochu, Don Soltman, Tom Legel, Terri Far, and Dan Klocko—are admired colleagues and friends with whom I am privileged to work.

The last 16 years would not have been possible without the support and tolerance of my chief executive officer, Joe Morris.

I want to express my gratitude to Janet Davis, Ed Avis, and Amanda Bove of Health Administration Press for their encouragement, guidance, and editorial expertise. They have contributed significantly to the final product.

Finally, but most importantly, I want to acknowledge my wife, Jean. She brings poetry into my world of prose, and she has been my guide, best friend, and inspiration as I seek to find my way in life's journey.

It is important to appreciate the biases that I bring to this work. I am essentially a traditionalist in attitude, someone who views his career in medicine as a vocational calling. I can still vividly recall my first day in medical school at the University of Rochester. I remember feeling excited, anxious, and scared, but, most of all, privileged as my new classmates and I toured Strong Memorial Hospital. I was going to become a doctor! Wow!

I contrast that day with the current state of affairs. Physicians frequently advise their children not to attend medical school, and they too often regret their own choices to have done so. What a transformation! This book represents my interpretation of why this transformation has occurred and what might be done to preserve the best of the historic traditions of medicine within the realities of a rapidly changing world of technological advancement and social and economic transformation.

My goal is to create opportunities for learning. In this book, I hope to provoke you, to cause you to expose your current operating assumptions and beliefs to assess whether they remain valid in light of new information. Unless you can imagine behaving differently, nothing will change. How you behave stems from your point of view. To behave differently demands that you change your point of view. That is my intention.

—Joseph S. Bujak, MD

CHAPTER 1

Understanding the Physician Culture

We started off trying to set up a small anarchist community,
but people wouldn't obey the rules.

—Alan Bennett[1]

EXPERT CULTURE VS. AFFILIATE CULTURE

Physicians are one example of an expert culture (Atchison and Bujak
2001). Engineers, architects, and lawyers in multi-specialty law
firms are other examples. Tenured professors at colleges and universities are an expert culture that is most analogous to physicians.
After achieving tenure, professors are beholden only to legal, professional, and ethical imperatives. Once medically licensed, physicians too are limited only by legal and ethical constraints. The
healthcare organization, however, has a "collective," or an "affiliate,"
culture. Understanding the expert culture of physicians and how it
differs from the culture of the healthcare organization helps to
explain many of the perceptual differences between the two that
cause tension and contribute to mistrust.

How Physicians Define Teamwork

An essential element of an expert culture is that experts make all decisions, issue by issue, from the perspective of how decisions will personally affect them. When I listen to physicians speak, I notice that they infrequently speak in the plural. Physicians usually say "I" and "me," but rarely "we" and "us." They do not have a collective identity. The transcendent value is individual autonomy.

Physicians' definition of teamwork is like the game of golf. Members of a golf team are seeded in a way that reflects their individual competency. The best member of the team is seeded number one. The next best member is seeded number two, and so on. When teams compete, the respective seeds compete against each other. Winning an individual match accrues points for the team, and, at the end of the day, the team that amasses the most points wins the competition. What, then, must an individual do to contribute to the likelihood that his team will win the competition? The answer is to win his individual match. If each member wins his individual match, the team wins. If the team loses, the members who have lost their individual matches are blamed. Teamwork to the physician is a zero-sum game in which the whole equals the sum of the parts.

This stands in great contrast to the affiliate culture of healthcare organizations. Teamwork within a healthcare organization is metaphorically equivalent to volleyball. The mantra of volleyball is "Dig! Set! Spike!" The roles of the team members are clear and interdependent. In this case, the whole can exceed the sum of its individual parts. The functionally best teams are not always comprised of the best individual players.

The physicians' and the healthcare organization's differing ideas of teamwork create tension within the healthcare community and are a reflection of acculturated differences that are, perhaps, reinforced by gender biases. That is, historically, physicians have been predominantly male, whereas nurses, who represent the largest demographic within the healthcare organization, have been predominantly female. Males are more inclined to be individualistic and competitive, whereas females are more inclined to collaborate (Gray 2004).

How Physicians Make Decisions

The difference between expert and affiliate cultures is also apparent in how decisions are made. The differing approach reflects the distinction between distributive justice and procedural justice (Kim and Mauborgne 1997). Physicians tend to focus on outcome. What matters most is that the outcome is successful. If the outcome is successful, how it was achieved is irrelevant because the end justifies the means. This is the essence of distributive justice. The affiliate culture of the healthcare organization, on the other hand, demands procedural justice. Procedural justice focuses on process. Individuals must feel that they have participated in the decision-making process in order for the outcome to be acceptable. A greater importance is placed on hearing individual opinions than on accepting them. Even if a solution is the right solution, it is unacceptable if it was decided without input from individuals. Put another way, if the process was inclusive, even the wrong outcome can be tolerated.

This time-consuming need to be inclusive drives physicians crazy. If you know the answer, just do it! Stop wasting time! According to the healthcare organization, however, imposing a decision without following the appropriate steps only ensures that the solution will be resisted. Any time that is saved initially will be spent later trying to create acceptance. Ironically, while physicians advocate for distributive justice when they are the ones giving the orders, they too demand procedural justice when others give orders to them.

What Motivates Physicians

Experts determine success by outperforming the competition. Achievement, taking risks, stamina, intense focus, quick decision making, and personal accountability are characteristic. Physicians are strongly vision or goal directed. They are not usually motivated by mission. Frequently, hospital administrators and their governing boards try to leverage the medical staff's behavior by suggesting that they have lost their professional "soul" because they do not to support the mission of the healthcare organization. However, the healthcare organization's mission is *its* mission and not the mission of the individual physicians. The critical challenge for the healthcare organization is to align the self-interest/goals of the individual physician with the needs of the organization. When a physician can see that supporting the goals of the healthcare organization serves her self-interest, then synergy occurs and magic can happen. When that vision is undeveloped, the individual physicians do not know where they fit with the future, so they tend to reproduce past behaviors and default to self-interest.

Why Physicians Do Not Collaborate

Healthcare is a culture of personal accountability in which the attending physicians bear the ultimate responsibility. In this context, one can quickly appreciate why physicians are taught to trust no one. In addition, physicians are usually highly competitive people; obtaining a medical degree is difficult without having been successfully competitive from an early age. Highly competitive people are predisposed not to trust. Competitive individuals are prone to see the world as a zero-sum game. If you win, I might lose. If your slice of the pie enlarges, mine might become smaller. Therefore, competitive individuals tend to hold their cards very close to their vests.

This has significant implications for healthcare organizations that seek to collaborate with physicians. All relationships are a form of negotiation. One can enter into negotiation by adopting one of four postures:

1. Competition (win/lose)
2. Accommodation (lose/win)

3. Compromise (lose/lose)
4. Collaboration (win/win)

Highly competitive physicians prefer to play a game of win/lose. When physicians face the possibility of losing in a game of win/lose, they invariably default to lose/lose, or compromise. Physicians typically find it very difficult to engage in potentially collaborative, or win/win, negotiations, because collaboration requires trust and highly competitive physicians are predisposed not to trust (Shell and Klasko 1997).

Physicians are also supremely self-confident. Because they are smart, they think they can do anything—without practice. I am convinced that any member of the medical staff believes that, if he so chooses, he could wake up tomorrow and do the job of the CEO better than she can—without practice. In physician training, "See one, do one, teach one" is frequently repeated. This attitude can foster a sense of arrogance and self-confidence that oversimplifies and underestimates the contributions of others who contribute to patient care. This is also one of the reasons why physicians do not listen well. The acculturated sense of omniscience and omnipotence helps to explain why physicians are quick to interrupt patients, draw conclusions, and act on initial impressions.

Physicians are expected to have all of the answers, bear the ultimate legal responsibility, and meet expectations of perfection. Therefore, it is not surprising that physicians have a strong need to be able to predict and thereby control their environments.

The Physician Approach to Problem Solving

The training of a physician is very hierarchical (Woods 2001). A physician progresses through training as one would ascend the rungs of a ladder. Because of accrued knowledge and experience, the physician then becomes a resource to those below. In this setting, it becomes culturally difficult to accept input from people perceived to be of a lower status. If you cannot express vulnerability, you cannot learn. That is, to learn you must be willing to acknowledge that your current state of knowing is either incomplete or inaccurate. For someone expected to have all of the answers, it becomes difficult, especially in public settings, to express that vulnerability.

Physicians are trained in the scientific method. Their approach to problem solving is deductive and linear. This approach is reinforced at the bedside, where physicians are under great pressure to act expeditiously to treat an acutely ill patient. This linear perspective stands in contrast to the systems perspective required of healthcare organization governance and administration. David Eddy has referred to this distinction as a problem of the apostrophe (Eddy 1998). Physicians are taught that they have an ethical imperative to serve as the *patient's* advocate. Short of doing harm, they are expected to do all that they can to benefit the patient, irrespective of the patient's ability to pay. Physicians advocate for each individual patient. Hospital administrators, on the other hand, are expected to serve as the *patients'* advocate. Hospital administrators recognize that a decision to allocate resources for one purpose precludes allocating those resources elsewhere. They are challenged to create the greatest good for the greatest number. Administrators advocate for all of the collective patients who need care. Each of these perspectives reflects an equally valid but separate set of ethics. No one can simultaneously apply both.

How Physicians View Time

The physician's sense of time is very different from that of a hospital administrator. What is "now" to a physician? In the healthcare setting, the word "stat" identifies actions that need to be done immediately. The word "now" to a physician means "without delay." What is "now" to a hospital administrator? If the frame of reference is capital allocations, "now" might be measured in terms of the next budget cycle. If a physician proposes a new opportunity to a hospital administrator, and the administrator agrees that the idea is good, then the physician expects to see it in place the next day. This distinctively different perception of time frequently causes tension and misunderstanding in the healthcare setting. Physicians really do not understand the delays, the frequent meetings, and the requirements for multiple consultations that often precede decision making within the healthcare organization. These time-consuming activities are in contrast to physician decision making in the service of individual patient needs in the acute care setting.

THE IMPORTANCE OF INDIVIDUAL AUTONOMY

Autonomy is the transcendent value within the physician community. A mutual commitment to the preservation of individual physician prerogative seems to be the only thing that unites physicians. If you ask for the opinion of the senior member of a physician group, he will gladly express his point of view. If you then ask him if he can speak on behalf of the group, he will invariably suggest that you talk to the other members individually. A physician is reluctant to speak on behalf of her colleagues, because she would resent her colleagues presuming to speak for her. This respect for individual physician autonomy also explains much of the difficulty physicians have in performing meaningful peer review.

Within an expert culture, where individual autonomy is the transcendent value and everyone is equal, how can one individual "lead" another? In such a culture, the presumption to lead is illegitimate. If a physician were to propose to his colleagues that he had the solution to a problem and that success would be assured if only they would follow him, their response would be the equivalent of, "So who died and left you boss?" Physicians will not interfere with an individual's right to go off in his own direction, but they would resent an expectation that they follow.

What is the most important requirement for being elected chief of the medical staff? It is that the person not be present when the nominations are made. The second most common rationale is that it is that person's turn to be stuck with the job. Being chief of staff is the equivalent of drawing the short straw. In my experience, when an individual physician actively seeks to be elected chief of the medical staff, she usually has a singular objective in mind—to have the chief executive officer (CEO) replaced. Leadership is made all the more difficult by the acculturated emphasis on independence and personal autonomy that all but precludes followership.

GENERATIONAL DIFFERENCES IN THE PHYSICIAN COMMUNITY

Traditionalist and Baby Boomer Physicians

Traditionalist physicians were born before 1945. For them, a career in medicine was a vocation, a response to a calling. Their self-identity and their professional identity are the same. They are physicians 24 hours a day, 365 days a year. Their primary motivation for becoming physicians was to have the respect that society accorded the unique role of healer. Motivation is intrinsic, and failure to live up to self-imposed expectations produces feelings of guilt. The physician and the physician's family often paid a significant price for this commitment. Physicians often missed too many dinners, school activities, and other significant events that are intrinsic to family life. The focus of the traditionalist physician is on professionalism and duty. Economic considerations are most often secondary or are assumed to accrue as a byproduct of a primary commitment to service.

Baby boomer physicians were similarly attracted to a career in medicine. They work very hard and appear on the surface to be quite similar to traditionalist physicians. However, baby boomers tend to primarily pursue status and the tangible rewards that often accompany higher status. In the course of their professional lives, professional respect began to erode with the advent of HMOs, increasing regulation, and shifting attitudes on the part of patients who no longer blindly accepted the physician's judgment. However, simultaneous with the advent of Medicare and Medicaid, as well as the widespread availability of employment-based health insurance, physicians' income began to increase significantly. Increasing income began to supersede respect as the primary reward for hard work.

Physicians are really products of the society from which they emerge. In my opinion, the traditionalist generation is trusting, hopeful, respectful, and loyal. The baby boomer generation is challenging, assertive, demanding, and far more critical.

Generation X Physicians

The character traits and cultural imperatives that emphasize autonomy and control generally apply to physicians who comprise either the traditionalist or the baby boomer generation. Generation X physicians are distinctly different from their older colleagues. If professionalism is the penultimate value for traditionalist and baby boomer physicians, Generation X physicians place a balanced life at the top of their value hierarchy. Being a physician is only part of their identity. They choose to be a physician on *their* terms. Unlike their predecessors, Generation X physicians have accumulated very significant debt in preparation for their professional career. Achieving security is very important to them. To control their time and to secure their expected income, they have significantly altered their choices of specialty practice. Very few are selecting a career in general surgery or general internal medicine, because managing time in these specialties is difficult. On the other hand, a surfeit of medical students select careers in dermatology, radiology, rehabilitation medicine, ophthalmology, and other primarily office-based specialties in which time can be managed and income expectations met.

Generation X physicians differ in a number of additional ways. In my experience, they do not value loyalty. In their minds, one should receive equal pay for equivalent competency. Rewarding longevity is foreign to their way of thinking. Having recently completed training, they often are more current and technically accomplished than their older colleagues. To their way of thinking, this proficiency should be rewarded and not subjugated to others who have "paid their dues." Generation X physicians are also more informal. For example, they dress more casually. They seek acknowledgment for substance over form—"Don't judge me for how I appear, judge me for the results of my work." Generation X physicians have little tolerance for wasting time. Attending meetings that accomplish nothing and participating in other citizenship-based activities that are traditional to medical-staff committee structures have no appeal to them.

Generation X physicians are disappearing from the hospital environment. Technological advances, progressive specialization, and lifestyle choices make it possible and desirable for younger physicians to practice independent of a hospital setting. Whereas the traditionalist and baby boomer physicians historically felt that covering the emergency department was part of their professional obligations and/or a way to build their practices, Generation X physicians strongly feel that they should be paid for serving that function. Primary care physicians from each generation are also removing themselves from the hospital. Changes in reimbursement and the cost of malpractice insurance now make it economically unfavorable for family practice physicians and general internists to practice obstetrics or assist in surgery on the one hand, or to manage the hospitalized patient on the other. For these reasons, generalists, upon whom specialists and healthcare organizations often depend for referrals, are no longer physically present in the hospital. Time is money.

Generation X physicians, unlike their predecessors, seek an employment model at the conclusion of their residency training. They have little appetite for joining private practice, where their reimbursement for similar work is often less than that received by their more senior colleagues. Serving an apprenticeship in pursuit of partnership is unacceptable. Moreover, the responsibilities that attend the management side of office practice would further encroach on time that they would prefer to allocate to other priorities. In my experience, Generation X physicians are primarily concerned with how little they have to work, how infrequently they would be on call, how much vacation they would receive, how much money they would earn, and how many additional perks they can negotiate. These expectations have relevance to physician recruitment. Manpower shortages have created a "seller's" market. Failure to meet the expectations of Generation X physicians removes your organization from consideration.

Older physicians carefully selected their practice opportunities often believing that they were a lifetime commitment. In contrast, Generation X physicians frequently change their practice locations. They do not often vocalize or negotiate around frustrations that they may experience in the workplace. The first indication an employer has that the Generation X physician is unhappy is often the receipt of a letter of resignation.

On the other hand, Generation X physicians bring significant positive contributions to the healthcare environment. They are very techno-savvy. They are more inclined to work interdependently and to delegate responsibility. (Leaving work by five o'clock is difficult without a willingness to delegate.) While they have no appetite for wasted work and wasted time, they are incredibly productive and willing to contribute when they can appreciate immediate and successful consequences. Generation X physicians seek to build their individual résumés. Their primary consideration is to enhance their value in the open marketplace.

So different are the attitudes and the value hierarchy of Generation X physicians that older physicians find it very difficult to align interests or to discover mutually acceptable solutions to challenging problems.

The Growing Number of Female Physicians

Another meaningful transition is consequent to the growing number of women in the physician workforce. Many medical school graduates are women. Having children significantly affects the amount of time that a female physician allocates to patient care activities. Working mothers often seek part-time employment or take long leaves of absence in deference to child rearing. For this reason female physicians are not as productive as male physicians. Hiring practices and the structure of work schedules often must accommodate these preferences.

DEALING WITH PHYSICIANS

It should be apparent from the previous sections that no individual in the physician community has signature authority. There is no one individual physician with whom an organization can negotiate who can commit others to honor the negotiation. There is no such thing as *physicians*. There is only *physician*. Dealing with physicians is a one-on-one sport.

Working with a Town-Hall Democracy

While preserving individual physician autonomy is the most important value in the physician community, when physicians are asked to make a collective decision, they paradoxically do so in the form of a "town-hall democracy"—one person, one vote, and majority rules. This has very significant implications. All groups act to defend the status quo. When an individual stands before their constituent group and proposes to shift one of their shared beliefs, in effect to change a paradigm, only about 15 percent of individuals in that group can imagine positive consequences. This minority segment is characterized by having tolerance for risk. While the exact percentage is debatable, all would agree that it is far less than 51 percent, which is the percentage of the group that must agree for any proposal to be accepted in the town-hall democracy. For this reason, the medical staff organization is always reactive. The medical staff organization is good at stalling initiatives, but it cannot act in a proactive, much less creative, fashion. For this reason, the medical staff organization represents an impotent vehicle for leading and managing transformational change.

Some of the cultural traits previously described further compromise decision making in the town-hall democracy. There are four primary avenues to decision making (Goleman, Boyatzis, and McKee 2002). The first type of decision making is delegated decision making. In this situation, because of acknowledged expertise, time pressures, or other considerations, someone within the organization either assumes or accepts the primary responsibility.

The second type is consultative decision making. In this circumstance, the person making the decision seeks input from a variety of other sources and considers that input to arrive at the "best" choice. This type of decision making frequently applies in the healthcare setting. Hospital administrators, when making decisions that might affect members of their medical staff, assess the opinions and the advice of various medical staff members. Herein is a dilemma. When the administrator asks the individual physician what she thinks of the proposed initiative, several consequences result:

1. Having asked the question, if the proposal is seen to have merit, the administrator accepts responsibility for creating the result.
2. The physician's contribution to creating that result ends with the advice given.
3. In asking many physicians for their opinions, the administrator is very likely to get many different recommendations. Since he cannot accept all of these recommendations and must choose the one that he feels is the best alternative, all those physicians whose advice was not heeded will conclude that the administrator

was acting in bad faith. They might say, "He asked for my advice and then did what he wanted to do anyway."

When engaging physicians in consultative decision making, communicate that you are seeking many different opinions, that you will consider all of the advice you receive, and that you will communicate your rationale after you have made a decision. In this way, you significantly avoid the misunderstandings that might otherwise result. Also, do not ask the physician, "What do you think of…?" but rather, "What could we do together to…?" This subtle change of words potentially accomplishes a meaningful shift in perception. When you ask a physician what she thinks, her answer becomes the sum and the substance of her total contribution to creating the result. Phrasing the inquiry in terms of what can be done together accomplishes two very important objectives:

1. The answer becomes more thoughtfully constructed.
2. The physician potentially commits her own energy and partici-
   pation in creating the future result.

A third type of decision making involves voting. Voting is an appropriate methodology in two circumstances:

1. When you have a long list that you want to shorten, vote on the items on the list. For example, if you have nine items on an agenda but only enough time to discuss three, you could vote on which of the nine to prioritize to fit the available time.
2. Vote when you have multiple alternatives, and no one is partic-
   ularly vested in any of them.

Managing for consensus is the fourth type of decision making. Achieving a decision through consensus requires negotiated give-and-take and a commitment to the time needed to agree on the final resolution. Achieving consensus is essential when multiple alternatives exist, when individuals are emotionally strongly vested in one or another of the alternatives, and when everyone will be expected to comply with the conclusions.

In the town-hall democracy of physician decision making, the following is an almost invariable scenario. The time-conscious physician defines a successful meeting as one that ends early. The issue presented is one that requires consensus decision making. Someone presents his preference and justification for his choice. Then another person advocates for her position and seeks to support her viewpoint. A third person then articulates for his selection. The discussion begins to go back and forth, with the meeting attendees debating the merits of each alternative. As the debate continues, someone in the back of the room (who is usually wearing scrubs) looks at *his* watch and notices that the time is ten minutes before the hour. He raises his hand and says, "We could talk about this until we are blue in the face and the cows come home. Let's just vote on it." Invariably, a vote follows. Those in the room whose strongly held preference was not selected leave the meeting totally uncommitted to the result and unwilling to behave accordingly. In my experience, this scenario plays out almost universally. Physicians are unwilling to allocate the time necessary to evolve a consensus decision, preferring instead to vote. Then they wonder why so many fail to comply with the behavior that is expected.

Respecting Individual Personality Differences

Like everyone else, physicians are distinguished by their individual personality preferences. Most readers are familiar with the Myers-Briggs personality profiles or other variations that seek to identify stylistic preferences for communicating and otherwise making sense of the environment. These preferences represent the triggers and the filters that individuals apply as they experience their environment. Individuals tend to selectively pay attention to those aspects of their environment that are most consistent with their existing way of making sense of the world and to weigh those elements in a disproportionately important way. Physicians very frequently choose their area of specialty practice as a reflection of their personality preferences. The action-oriented decider might choose to become a surgeon or an emergency department physician. Those with a preference for organizing skills might seek a career in pathology or neurology, in which structure and function are strongly correlated. Big-picture thinkers who like to strategize might be drawn toward careers in diagnostic medicine, oncology, or infectious diseases, in which the breadth of possibilities requires a capacity to synthesize across many different domains. Those individuals who are more sensitive to relationships might select pediatrics, psychiatry, primary care, or obstetrics—specialties more consistent with their intrinsic affinities. Is there any wonder that there is no such thing as *physicians*?

DEVELOPING PHYSICIAN LEADERS

Healthcare organizations recognize the importance of identifying physician leaders and investing in their leadership potential. Significant challenges confront the potential physician leader. As discussed, leadership in the physician community is seen as illegitimate. Moreover, cultural and selection biases confront those physicians who are willing to assume such a role. Physicians are predisposed to a linear view and are not used to appreciating the complexities that attend managing a healthcare organization. The ability to achieve a systems perspective requires that the would-be physician leader be a good listener who is willing to suspend judgment. No meaningful change occurs outside of conversation (Shaw 2002). Indeed, shared meaning is the birthplace of synergy. The clinical decision maker is used to a more activist approach.

Moving from positions of informal leadership to positions of formal leadership within the organization is a transformative journey. Those who rise to positions of informal leadership do so because they are eloquent spokespersons for the shared needs of their constituency. However, when moving into positions of formal leadership, the individual can never again be "one of the boys" (Malone 1983). For formal leaders, the mission of the organization must supersede the needs of any one individual. As physician leaders begin to acquire a systems perspective, appreciate the organizational complexities, and recognize the laws of unintended consequences, they also begin to apply a vocabulary and share a perspective that is foreign to the narrow self-interest of their former constituents who, at that point, reject them as having gone over to "the dark side."

When physician leaders seek to resolve organizational issues as a clinician, they encounter significant resistance. Physicians are problem solvers. They want to fix things immediately and have little tolerance for delay. However, too often the immediate and short-term fixes become the sources of tomorrow's problems. This tendency toward wanting to aggressively fix things often results in workarounds that invariably add complexity and increased variation, as well as produce waste and potentially compromise patient safety and clinical quality of care. Moreover, aggressiveness in an inherently slow-moving system creates instability (Senge 1990). Physicians who are used to putting out fires now must focus on building fire stations. In this context, the impatient physician leader pursues distributive justice, only to have their proposal rejected by those who would be affected by the change because they were not included on the decision-making process.

Daniel Goleman and his colleagues (2002) have described six leadership styles. Four of these leadership styles are well received. These include visionary, coaching, democratic, and affiliate leadership styles. Two styles, the command style and the pace-setting style, create dissonance. Physician culture predisposes physicians to apply the latter two styles of leadership, because physicians are used to giving orders and acting rapidly and independently.

I personally believe that the only way to encourage people to commit to new behaviors is by allowing them to connect the dots between the new information and the implications of that information for their own behavior. They must discover for themselves how new behaviors can better serve their self-interest in light of new information. This can only be done in small-group dialogue. The ability to bring physicians together for an opportunity to sustain that dialogue is a huge challenge. Physicians are usually unwilling to commit time to the possibility of discovering new solutions. Sometimes, physicians seem to prefer to complain and sustain current and ineffective behaviors rather than pause for the opportunity to discover new approaches.

Administrators often ask the question, "Should the physician leader continue in clinical practice?" The assumption here is that continuing to see patients will sustain credibility among clinical colleagues. In my view, the skill sets that support performance excellence for the physician leader are distinct and require a dedication similar to those that would support clinical excellence. As mentioned previously, as soon as the physician leader adopts a systems perspective and begins to appreciate organizational complexity, he begins to validate positions articulated by the administrative staff causing his colleagues to reject him. This occurs regardless of whether the physician leaders continue to practice. In my view, then, if the physician leader chooses to maintain a clinical presence, it should be because it gives him distinct and personal pleasure and not because it will support credibility among his physician colleagues.

WHY MANAGING PHYSICIAN RELATIONSHIPS IS SO DIFFICULT

It should be obvious by now that a prescriptive or unified approach to managing physician relationships does not exist. The physician community behaves as an expert culture and additionally represents a complex matrix of generational differences, preferred styles of relating that are often reflected in choice of specialty practice, and gender differences. These are compounded by an overriding commitment to respecting individual physician autonomy.

How, then, does governance and hospital administration access physician opinion? Where do they seek advice that could guide strategic decision making as it relates to partnering with physicians?

Which physicians are most inclined to participate in either governance or administrative activities? Traditionalist and baby boomer physicians are far more likely to have the time and the inclination to participate. Following their advice, however, is likely to lead to proposals that are totally unacceptable to Generation X physicians. Advice from Generation X physicians would similarly be unacceptable to older physicians.

Too often, those in positions of governance or administration within healthcare organizations assume that employment is one way to influence and/or control the behavior of physicians. While the terms of monetary reimbursement contained within the physician's employment contract influences specific behaviors, a commitment to individual professional autonomy transcends employment status and renders the term "employed physician" an oxymoron. Physicians predominantly respond to clinical context and are less influenced by economic or regulatory imperatives. Patient care and self-interest trump all other considerations, and often the two are in conflict with each other and create tension for the individual physician.

SUMMARY

There is no such thing as *physicians*. The medical staff represents an impotent vehicle for leading and managing change, and any physician strategy must be pluralistic and robust. Because all groups act to sustain the status quo and because physicians make collective decisions in the format of a town-hall democracy, you must be willing to lead to critical mass and not to consensus.

NOTE

1. Quoted in Mardy Grothe, *Oxymoronica: Paradoxical Wit and Wisdom from History's Greatest Wordsmiths* (New York: HarperCollins, 2004), 24.

REFERENCES

Atchison, T., and J. Bujak. 2001. *Leading Transformational Change: The Physician-Executive Partnership*. Chicago: Health Administration Press.

Eddy, D. 1998. Presentation on physician leadership to VHA's Physician Leadership Council, Dallas, TX, May 22.

Goleman, D., R. Boyatzis, and A. McKee. 2002. *Primal Leadership: Realizing the Power of Emotional Intelligence*. Boston: Harvard Business School Press.

Gray, J. 2004. *Men Are from Mars, Women Are from Venus: The Classic Guide to Understanding the Opposite Sex*. New York: Harper Collins.

Kim, W. C., and R. Mauborgne. 1997. "Fair Process: Managing in the Knowledge Economy." *Harvard Business Review* 75 (4): 65–75.

Malone, D. M. 1983. *Small Unit Leadership: A Commonsense Approach*. Novato, CA: Presidio Press.

Senge, P. 1990. *The Fifth Disciple*. New York: Doubleday.

Shaw, P. 2002. *Changing Conversations in Organizations: A Complexity Approach to Change*. London: Routledge.

Shell, G. R., and S. K. Klasko. 1996. "Negotiating: Biases Physicians Bring to the Table." *Physician Executive* 22 (12): 4–7.

Woods, M. 2001. *Applying Personal Leadership Principles to Health Care: The DEPO Principle*. Tampa, FL: American College of Physician Executives.

CHAPTER 2

Physician Response to Forces that Are Transforming the Provider Community

Our dilemma is that we hate change and love it at the same time; what we really want is for things to remain the same but get better.

—Sydney J. Harris[1]

TRANSFORMATIONAL FORCES

A number of dynamic forces are transforming our current health-care system. Some of these forces include technology, research, and rising costs; patient needs and expectations; progressive subspecialization; access to healthcare; pay-for-performance initiatives; and growing physician dissatisfaction.

Technology, Research, and Rising Costs

As a culture, the United States is technologically dependent. We seek to find technological solutions to our most pressing problems (Annas 1996). Technological and pharmaceutical innovations fuel growing expectations and contribute to the rising costs of healthcare.

The government has significantly reduced funding of basic research through National Institutes of Health grants. Because of this, pharmaceutical and technology firms are providing an increasing proportion of funding for research. These for-profit entities expect significant returns on investment. Direct-to-consumer advertising moves research from discovery to entitlement in a very short period. Most new technology comes with a significant price tag, and these diagnostic and therapeutic innovations are often applied before their appropriateness is determined.

Members of the physician community are often co-opted by this process. Physicians dedicated to research become dependent on funding from for-profit agencies. The source of funding has a stake in what is studied, how it is studied, and whether the results are published. Peer reviewers are often financially related to the sponsoring organization, and the journals are dependent on advertising revenue that is provided by the same companies. Therefore, what passes for peer-reviewed and evidence-based medical practice is strongly influenced by the profit motives of the sponsoring companies.

Physicians who are involved in research, or who are in other ways economically supported by for-profit companies, become the providers of "continuing medical education" as they travel the country to promote the latest intervention. Joint ownership of specialty hospitals, ambulatory surgery centers, and diagnostic imaging centers is often evidence of physician partnerships with venture capital. Manufacturers of implant devices often "partner" with physicians in the promotion of the widespread utilization of their product. The application and use of technology are growing, often in the absence of definitive evidence of clinical benefit, as is the case with some cardiac pacemakers and devices used in back surgery.

The dependence on technology and its promotion by companies that have a vested interest in its application have perhaps caused society to view death as an optional event. Individuals want access to any intervention that might conceivably benefit them, and yet they expect to pay little or nothing. Society has too little personal accountability for the consequences of lifestyle choices and an undue reliance on last-minute fixes provided by the healthcare safety net. Moreover, society expects healthcare to be perfect in its application.

The malpractice crisis certainly has played a role in the excessive application of medical resources. This crisis has significantly affected access to certain medical specialties in states where premiums have become inordinately high. In many communities, obstetricians, neurosurgeons, and trauma services are difficult to access because of demographic shifts within the provider community due to the malpractice climate. It isn't surprising that many trained neurosurgeons are restricting their practice to spine surgery, preferring to avoid cranial surgery. The former is highly lucrative, while the latter is frequently attended by enhanced threats of malpractice litigation.

Overhead for practicing physicians continues to increase. Wages, benefits, and the costs of supplies and utilities are increasing. Overhead related to satisfying the demands of the payer and regulatory communities and the high cost of malpractice insurance are additionally burdensome. The margin per unit of service is shrinking. Healthcare payers have observed that physicians sometimes adjust their practice to achieve an expected level of income; this phenomenon has been called "the target income principle." Since the profit margin per unit of service rendered is shrinking, and given that physicians consciously or unconsciously seek to attain a targeted level of income, physicians have changed their behavior to allow them to perform an increasing number of units of service within a given period.

Patient Needs and Expectations

Our healthcare system is currently designed around an acute care model. When an individual is acutely ill, he requires access to doctors and hospitals. However, the majority of current encounters with the healthcare system are not for acute illness, but rather for services related to chronic disease or wellness. When a patient is chronically ill or seeking to remain healthy, she requires access to information rather than access to doctors and hospitals.

The increase in medical knowledge has reached a point that the number of potential variables that attend a given patient problem exceeds the capacity of the human mind to manage or integrate them. Historically, patients relied on their physician to gather information, make decisions, and intervene on their behalf. The patient was relatively ignorant and dependent on the physician. Today, especially with access to the Internet, patients present to their physician armed with more information than the physician can possibly recall. The role of the physician is transforming into interpreter of information and adviser to patients who progressively seek to be partners in the decision making that affects their health and welfare.

The changing focus on managing chronic disease and maintaining wellness is significantly influencing medical economics. I have heard it said that more money is spent on nontraditional healthcare interventions than on allopathic primary care services. Most of this money would be out of pocket and retail. The growing use of physician extenders, the development of concierge medicine, and the expansion of services available via the Internet are examples of this.

The digitalization of healthcare information empowers the individual to seek consultative advice and/or therapeutic intervention from providers who are far away, which significantly challenges the protective affect of licensure. Telemedicine, robotic surgery, and the accessibility of prescription medications dispensed by providers from distant locations are other examples of patient empowerment. Organizations like the Cleveland Clinic, the Mayo Clinic, and certain cancer treatment facilities advertise nationally and internationally and maintain patient education resources on their frequently accessed Internet sites.

In virtually all industries, the needs of the customer are the greatest concern. Education and healthcare appear to be two significant exceptions. Universities are primarily about teachers and not students. Healthcare is more about providers than patients. The way healthcare is organized and delivered usually defers to the convenience and the needs of the providers. If healthcare providers were truly focused on the needs of the patients, they would not dress them as they do, feed them as they do, make them wait the way they do, or address them in a language that they cannot understand. Healthcare providers awaken patients in the early morning hours so that their laboratory results are ready when the physician rounds. Healthcare providers ask patients to report for elective surgery very early in the morning, even though the start time for the case might be closer to noon, while requiring them not to eat or drink anything. Too often, patients' families are kept in the dark as the busy physician runs from place to place in deference to a progressively crowded schedule. People crowd emergency department waiting rooms because the emergency department has become the physician's surrogate. Veterinarians and dentists have better adapted to changing service expectations than have most physicians.

The growing emphasis on patient satisfaction surveys and the soon-to-be publicly reported results of those surveys are slowly transforming this behavior. Consumer driven healthcare with rising co-payments and deductibles reinforces this trend.

Because patients who are active in their care can now access health-related information, the physician's role has transitioned from one of being knowledge gatherer and decider to being organizer and translator. Whereas historically the physician knew everything and the patient knew nothing, placing the physician in a position of absolute power, the patient now has access to more information than the physician can recall, which shifts the balance of power and transforms the relationship. Couple this with progressive specialization, generational shifts in attitude and value hierarchy, a growing reliance on technology, and the imposed application of what currently passes for evidence-based medicine, and we have a situation in which the science of medicine has transcended the art. Curing has displaced healing, and the physician has become the gatekeeper to technology.

In my view, both the physician and the patient are being short-changed in the process. Progressive specialization, growing complexity, economic pressures, changing expectations, decreasing reimbursements, the malpractice climate, the growing influence of pharmaceutical and technology firms, and the absence of ethical imperatives are all resulting in the deprofessionalization of medicine.

Progressive Subspecialization

Progressive subspecialization is significantly transforming how healthcare services are provided. Physicians are focusing more narrowly. In part, this reflects the growing complexity within medicine. In addition, physicians can reduce their risk, increase their income, and control their lifestyle by narrowing their focus.

Medical sub-specialists are still required to pass general internal medicine boards. They then progress through subspecialty training and become boarded in their medical subspecialty. Subspecialists may then progress to further refinements in their training by accepting fellowships in a more focused area within their subspecialty. The specialty of cardiology and the cardiology subspecialty of electrophysiology are examples. Electrophysiologists restrict practice to cardiac electrophysiology and no longer involve themselves in the care of general cardiac disease, much less illnesses that are in the domain of general internal medicine.

Orthopedics is another example. An orthopedist used to be just an orthopedist. Now, orthopedists frequently restrict practice to hip or knee replacement; arthroscopy; the hand, shoulder, foot, or back; or trauma. How do you construct an orthopedic on-call schedule? Do you want someone who specializes in hand or back surgery to manage a fractured femur? The specialist in question may no longer feel competent to treat fractures and has no interest in doing so. As a patient, who would you want to manage your fracture?

Access to Healthcare

Physician access is becoming a very significant issue in American medicine. Changing demographics, increasing demand, reductions in physician manpower, and the progressively increasing number of people without health insurance are just some of the factors contributing to the problem of access. In many communities, newly arrived residents can have difficulty finding physicians who are accepting new patients, especially if the payer source is governmental. Given the shortage of generalists and the reluctance of specialty physicians to address issues outside of their restricted areas of practice, patients are often left to negotiate a merry-go-round of referrals, if they are lucky enough to secure appointments in the first place.

Pay-for-Performance Initiatives

Pay for performance is a growing phenomenon. Payers, regulators, and organizations devoted to improving patient safety and clinical quality are demanding that clinicians provide process and/or outcome data that patients can use to decide which providers they prefer to see. The clinicians whose data suggests they are more effective and/or efficient are "rewarded" by being included in preferred provider panels or by receiving increased reimbursement for services provided. Paying someone more for doing the right thing, while continuing to pay others the going rate for substandard performance, strikes me as unethical. More and more, this is evolving into "we won't pay if you fail to perform." Meanwhile, the need to provide the data used to profile physician practice requires ever more sophisticated information technology systems, which further drive up costs in terms of software, hardware, and the personnel required to enter, process, and report the data.

Frequently, physicians find themselves at odds with payers. While payers seek to maximize their medical loss ratio, physicians pursue progressive diagnostics in response to their fear of malpractice litigation and increasing patient expectations. Healthcare providers, in contrast to most other industries, have a distorted definition of economic value. To most providers, fair reimbursement is the cost of what it took to provide the service, plus a reasonable additional amount for profit. Healthcare providers fail to appreciate that value is really defined by what someone is willing to pay to access the product or service. It is analogous to valuing real estate. You can know to the penny what it cost you to build your home, but your house is only worth what someone else is willing to pay for it.

New business models and an increasing number of midlevel and alternative medicine providers are challenging the traditional role of the primary care physician. Eye surgery has become commoditized, and accessing prescriptions through the Internet has disrupted traditional relationships.

As the costs for healthcare continued to climb, and as payers became progressively more aware of the variation that accompanies medical decision making, it was inevitable that payers would insist on better ways of ensuring that they get what they pay for. Payers have been requesting data that justifies the costs incurred. In addition, they are seeking data that reflects the quality of the outcome. They have expectations that the credentialing and privileging process be adequately supported by quality peer review. Historically, the provider community responded by saying, "Trust us, it's too complicated." As costs continued to rise and as providers continued to resist requests for data, payers began to look to third-party intermediaries to carry out the oversight function. The health maintenance organization (HMO) resulted.

A willingness to hold peers responsible to a level of performance that is above the legally required minimum is a condition that accompanies professional status (O'Conner and Lanning 1992). The physician culture, with its emphasis on the primacy of individual physician autonomy, finds it difficult to exercise this responsibility. This has contributed to the deprofessionalization of medicine and to an erosion of trust and respect. Physicians have lost significant authority in the decision-making process that accompanies individual patient care.

Growing Physician Dissatisfaction

Challenges to the physicians' primary place in the healthcare system have significantly eroded their morale. Physicians too frequently advise their children against going to medical school and often resent their own choice to have done so. Physicians list the following factors as reasons for their eroding morale:

- Loss of autonomy
- Bureaucratic red tape
- Patient overload
- Low reimbursement
- Loss of respect
- Medical malpractice environment

Insurers, regulators, payers, utilization review nurses, legislators, and judges are now making decisions once historically under the sole control of the physician. Paperwork is a nightmare. Most physician offices employ two or more full-time equivalents just to comply with the needs of insurers and regulators. Simply trying to keep straight different payer formularies is a huge headache. As mentioned previously, in an attempt to protect yearly income in a climate where each unit of service is accompanied by a shrinking margin, physicians have begun to work ever harder. The malpractice environment creates a situation where the patient and the physician often see each other as potential adversaries.

As care becomes progressively depersonalized, as relationships give way to technology, and as patient expectations escalate, physicians experience a loss of respect. Physicians historically were among the most trusted individuals in society, but now they are often viewed with suspicion. Some patients worry that the doctor's decision making may be self-serving. Patients trust nurses more than they do physicians.

OVERCOMING THE CHALLENGES

Physicians are seeking ways to bolster their falling income and to identify sources of capital. Healthcare organizations represent a potential source of that capital. However, when the physician looks at the healthcare organization as a potential source of capital, she sees an organization that has large fixed costs, an unfavorable payer mix, and the seeming inability to make timely decisions (Zismer 2004). At the same time, the healthcare organization is fully aware that it cannot be successful without partnering with members of its medical staff. Outdated and limiting beliefs have compromised attempts by the healthcare organization to collaborate with physicians. Healthcare organizations fail to realize that

- hospitals and physicians are not in the same business,
- when competing with venture capital for physician allegiance, the pure not-for-profit business model no longer suffices;
- the medical staff is not an economic entity; and
- the healthcare organization must treat physicians equitably and not equally to succeed.

Healthcare organizations are further hampered by a desire to integrate patient care in a world that is becoming progressively more subspecialized. Indeed, how to simultaneously integrate and specialize is one of the great challenges confronting traditional healthcare organizations. Though many stakeholder groups emphasize the importance of integrating patient care, if reimbursement is any yardstick, no one values the integration function. Creation of the electronic health record is considered the key that will accomplish this integration function, but someone will have to read that record and provide the appropriate oversight function.

Another major challenge is whether healthcare organizations should elect to "stick to their knitting"—to continue to confine themselves to their core competency of providing care in an acute model of disease—or to venture into the world of retail medicine. Retail medicine captures discretionary out-of-pocket spending absent regulatory oversight.

I define retail medicine as any service for which no reimbursement code has been created, including

- alternative healthcare;
- diagnostics;
- wellness;
- health maintenance;
- cosmetic surgery;
- elective interventions such as massage and aromatherapy; and
- dcupuncture.

As costs escalate in the rendering of acute care medicine in the high-tech world of the hospital, and as reimbursement fails to keep pace with those incremental costs, positive operating margins become progressively more difficult to achieve. In addition, increasing regulatory requirements represent unfunded mandates that further compromise the operating margin. Not only are additional employees needed, but also the amount of time that bedside caregivers are distracted from direct contact with their patients is progressively increasing as they are required to comply with burdensome documentation. I project that margins in the delivery of wholesale healthcare will continue to shrink and that economic viability will continue to migrate to ambulatory-based retail services.

The traditional healthcare organization is not skilled in the understanding and management of nontraditional acute care products and services. As we will see later, technology is progressively driving the locus of healthcare delivery closer to the patient's home and is continuingly reducing the training and skill required to apply that intervention to the point that self-care is becoming a reality.

The doubling time of knowledge is currently estimated to be somewhere between three and four years. Indeed, the progression of technology and knowledge is advancing faster than the traditional four-year curriculum of formal medical school training. By the time a physician finishes medical training, much of what he learned will have become outdated or incorrect. This is especially problematic for the physician who has completed formal training. Technological advances render historic ways of delivering care less acceptable and require that the physician stays current. In the physician community, there is an often-repeated dictum that new skills are acquired through "See one, do one, teach one." This challenges governing boards that must extend privileges. What represents an adequate demonstration of competency as it applies to the learning of new techniques or to the application of new interventions for the older physician? Patients are additionally at a disadvantage in their attempts to judge physician competency when those services are rendered in an ambulatory setting, where no privileging body has oversight control.

TRANSFORMING HEALTHCARE DELIVERY

Healthcare Trends

How will robotics, genomics, proteomics, nanotechnology, and telemedicine affect the traditional delivery of healthcare services? Physicians feel threatened by the accelerating pace of change. Joe Flower (2006), a healthcare futurist, has addressed seven major trends that are going to significantly transform current healthcare delivery, sooner rather than later:

1. Major disease categories, including cancer and cardiovascular disease, will be controllable.
2. There will be a shift toward pharmaceutical intervention.
3. Surgery will occur less often and be performed less invasively.
4. The resurgence of infectious diseases and drug-resistant organisms will cause major challenges.
5. Diagnostic procedures that approach absolute certainty will be developed.
6. Digitalized healthcare will create a data repository so large that questions as to the most successful approach to a given disease or problem will be answered with statistically guided precision.
7. Healthcare delivery sites will polarize.

Quaternary care will be delivered in academic centers where major technological breakthroughs will be discovered, and less complicated care will be provided in ambulatory-based community centers. Flower (2006) expresses concern for the viability of the traditional secondary and tertiary care sites that are so prevalent today because of the affect of the trends described.

Focus Factories

Focus factories (Herzlinger 1997) are an example of how specialization, economics, and changing expectations are transforming the medical landscape. Ambulatory surgery centers could be considered an example of a focus factory. In this setting, elective surgery is efficiently performed in ways that meet and usually exceed patient expectations. In addition, operational efficiencies often allow a surgeon, for example, to perform five surgical operations in the time required to perform three in the traditional hospital operating room. The economic advantage to the surgeon is the ability to operate on two additional patients in the same amount of time. That profitability far exceeds the investment returns from having an ownership position in the same ambulatory surgical center.

Even more focused are the efficiencies obtained when only a single procedure is performed in a high-volume setting. This occurs in ophthalmology when treating cataracts or performing Lasik surgery. A clinic in Toronto only does hernia surgery, a clinic in Minneapolis only performs back surgery, and there are many endoscopy centers across the country. The ability to standardize processes creates enhanced efficiency, effectiveness, and quality of patient experience. Additionally, physicians feel they have control over when they operate and who assists them in surgery. These benefits are often absent in hospital operating rooms, where the organization must be prepared to deal with emergency situations, anesthesia may be less efficient, or the surgeon performing the preceding case unusually slow.

Disruptive Technologies

Disruptive technologies (Christensen 1997) are another example of transformations to the current delivery of healthcare. Technological advances in diagnostics and therapeutics are invariably more expensive than the technologies that preceded them. These innovations are labeled "sustaining technologies" in that they command high reimbursement, are universally seen as desirable advances, and are appealing to the mainstream market.

To recoup the cost of the new technology, the expense is applied to all patients in situations for which the technology has potential application. Yet, pre-existing technologies are rarely abandoned in deference to the more expensive and more sophisticated new technology. Early on, the new technology is applied in addition to, rather than instead of, the older, less sophisticated interventions, which adds to the cost of care. However, each new technology enhances diagnostic precision by a progressively smaller percentage. That is, in the pursuit of diagnostic certainty, more sophisticated technologies have utility in an ever-shrinking percentage of patients who present with a given diagnostic entity. The incremental cost of procedures that potentially benefit fewer patients means that most patients are unnecessarily "over served." They could have been successfully diagnosed or effectively treated by less expensive interventions.

As patients become responsible for paying a progressively increasing share of the cost of their care, they become more discerning in their willingness to accept recommended interventions. In this setting, healthcare begins to act more like a traditional market. If you tell a patient that you are 97 percent sure that the diagnosis is correct, but that you could become 2 percentage points more certain by the application of a technology that would personally cost him an additional $2,000, the likelihood that he will proceed becomes critically dependent on the amount of his disposable income. When all healthcare costs are borne by a third party, as long as the new intervention is without significant risk, why would the patient not opt for the additional level of diagnostic precision? This creates an opportunity for the emergence of a disruptive technology.

Disruptive technologies are distinguished from sustaining technologies in the following ways. As stated, sustaining technologies are high-cost, high-tech enhancements over currently existing technology. They represent significant embellishments, have high margins, and are highly desired by patients, traditional payers, and practitioners who desire to remain on the cutting edge. Disruptive technologies, on the other hand, typically have low margins, appeal to a small market segment, are not desired by traditional payers, utilize inferior technology, and are so new as to not be able to support a business plan. In effect, in the high-tech world of healthcare organizations, these disruptive technologies appear inferior and unappealing.

An example of a disruptive technology that has become mainstream is urgent care centers, which seem primitive, understaffed, and in other ways inferior to the high-tech emergency departments that are staffed by board-certified emergency physicians and trauma surgeons. However, these businesses are cash or cash equivalent only, provide immediate access to the caregiver, significantly reduce waiting times, and siphon off a meaningful source of revenue from the traditional emergency department that is busy caring for the injured motorcyclist with no health insurance. Other examples of disruptive technologies include

- home pregnancy tests;
- self-administered rapid strep screening kits;
- acupuncture;
- massage therapy; and
- midwives.

Each one of these technologically inferior, less expensive, and more convenient disruptive technologies cuts out the traditional provider.

Disruptive technology creates both threat and opportunity. For example, let us examine a situation that confronts the primary care physician. The advent of nurse practitioners represented a significant threat to the primary care physician as the point of entry for healthcare services. Physicians initially resisted the licensing of nurse practitioners, seeking to limit the depth and breadth of services they could provide and originally requiring them to work only under the auspices of a licensed physician.

However, rural areas that are typically underserved by physicians had unmet needs for access to healthcare services. This need politically overrode physicians' objections and led to an ever-expanding independence for nurse practitioners, especially in rural settings. Once nurse practitioners became potentially independent, primary care physicians discovered an opportunity that resulted from this disruption to their preexisting dominant position. Instead of resisting their presence, many physicians employed one or more nurse practitioners, because they unburden the primary care physician by seeing patients with uncomplicated illnesses or wellness needs. The supervising physicians can bill his standard fee while paying the nurse practitioner a salary. This has created an income opportunity for the primary care physician who stopped seeing the nurse practitioner as a threat and began to see this disruptive technology as an opportunity to change his business model.

This entire process is called "moving down-market." Instead of viewing less-trained people as competitors, physicians co-opted the process by incorporating and applying nurse practitioners into their business models.

Simultaneously, the primary care physician can take advantage of technology to allow her to "move up-market" and co-opt procedures that historically could only be performed by physicians with specialty training. Today, many primary care physicians are doing various forms of gastrointestinal endoscopies in their offices, performing bone densitometry, doing exercise cardiac stress testing, and providing other services that historically were reserved for specialists.

Various types of providers are consolidating in order to service a broader range of related patient care needs. Historically, ophthalmologists saw optometrists as inferiorly trained interlopers. As ophthalmologists' income declined, this attitude changed. Now ophthalmologists and optometrists frequently practice together in the same business enterprise, often incorporating opticians as well, and cover the entire spectrum of eye-related concerns. All of the participants spend the day doing what they have been trained to do. The optometrist does normal eye exams and refractions, referring abnormal findings for evaluation by the ophthalmologist, who spends most of her day in the operating room. This puts both of their special training to the best use, and both benefit from having the optician dispense eyeglasses and contact lenses. The integrated enterprise is beneficial to each component.

The same dynamic applies to the relationship of orthopedists to chiropractors and physical therapists. Instead of demeaning each other, they now join to service the entire range of back pain. The orthopedist spends his day in the operating room, while the chiropractor spends the day dealing with nonoperative back pain. Both utilize the services of the physical therapist in dealing with issues of rehabilitation. All benefit from the integration.

SUMMARY

Technology and knowledge are expanding at an ever-accelerating rate. Success is critically tied to the ability to adapt. As patients bear an increasing responsibility to finance their own healthcare needs, they will become more discerning in their evaluation of the acceptability of suggested diagnostic and therapeutic interventions. Disruptive technologies will continue to push the locus of care and the skill of the individual who applies the technology closer to the patient's home and to the patient. The physician, who was the collector of information and decision maker on behalf of his patients, has now become an organizer, an interpreter, and a partner in decision making as he advises patients who seek to become partners in the management of their own health and welfare.

Every physician will be confronted with threats to her current position by economic forces, advancing technology, changing patient expectations, and the need to remain knowledgeable in a world where the doubling time of knowledge is approaching three years. Sustainability is clearly tied to adaptability. Technology will change, relationships will change, and economics will change. This is true of all professions and all industries. Physicians cannot hide behind licensure and will progressively be required to document competency by providing data in support of their practice efficiency, effectiveness, and quality of service.

NOTE

1. Quoted in Mardy Grothe, *Oxymoronica: Paradoxical Wit and Wisdom from History's Greatest Wordsmiths* (New York: HarperCollins, 2004), 44.

REFERENCES

Annas, G. J. 1996. "Toward Ecology of Health: Beyond the Military and Market Metaphors." *Healthcare Forum Journal* 39 (30): 30–4.

Christensen, C. 1997. *The Innovator's Dilemma.* Boston: Harvard School Press.

Flower, J. 2006. "Health Futures." Presentation to Carolinas Health System. Charlotte, NC, September.

Herzlinger, R. 1997. *Market-Driven Healthcare: Who Wins, Who Loses in the Transformation of America's Largest Service Industry.* Reading, PA: Addison-Wesley Publishing.

O'Conner, S. J., and J. A. Lanning. 1992. "The End of Autonomy? Reflections on the Post Professional Physician." *Healthcare Management Review* 17 (1): 63–72.

Zismer, D. 2004. "Hospital-Physician Relationships." Presentation to VHA Southwest, Scottsdale, AZ, May.

CHAPTER 3

Specific Approaches to Influencing Physician Behavior

It is a profitable thing, if one is wise, to seem foolish.
—Aeschylus, in *Prometheus Bound*[1]

BUILD TRANSFORMATIONAL EXPERIENCES AND ESTABLISH TRUST

Trust is the foundation on which all relationships are based. One of the reasons trust is essential is somewhat counterintuitive. Without trust, a relationship cannot sustain a healthy conflict of ideas (Lencioni 2002). Trust increases in proportion to the frequency of meaningful interactions. A willingness to express vulnerability is essential to establishing trust. This occurs when you allow others to know you outside the formality of your professional role.

If you have ever been in a conversation about a troublesome emotional experience, either as the attentive listener or the speaker, you will know what I mean. At the conclusion of this conversation, the relationship is never the same. A sense of closeness and appreciation results from this connection. An aphorism states, "It is impossible to hate someone whose story you know."

A willingness to reveal your frustrations, to admit mistakes, to ask for assistance, and to share your vulnerabilities is an integral component of building transformational relationships and establishing trust.

Engaging in personal conversation for 4½ hours while in a golf cart can do more to establish a sense of trust than having superficial conversations in the hallway for 4½ years. Building physician relationships requires the time and the effort of engaging in meaningful one-on-one conversation. Allowing the physician to appreciate who you are outside the pre-existing assumptions that accompany their interpretation of your professional role is essential to establishing trusting and enduring relationships.

Meaningful change does not occur outside of conversation (Shaw 2002). The dialectic that is experienced in conversations that address a meaningful conflict of ideas is the birthplace of synergy. This healthy conflict of ideas cannot occur in an environment that lacks trust.

ENCOURAGE SELF-DISCOVERY AND SELF-INTEREST

The most effective way to influence another's behavior is by nurturing self-discovery. You cannot teach a person anything. You can only help him discover it for himself. Self-discovery—the ability to make sense of new information or to personally reconnect the dots—accompanies the "Aha!" that can occur in open dialogue about subjects of personal importance. Self-discovery is how adults learn and is the most effective way to influence physician behavior.

The dynamic occurs as follows. Five to seven individuals who are involved in creating something meaningful together sit around a table to discuss the relevance of new information related to the work in question. A facilitator introduces new information or new data. The facilitator then encourages the group to discuss the relevance or implications of this new information. How might the new information affect their behavior? The sharing of individual responses in conversation allows the group to begin to collectively make sense of what is happening. This is the most effective way to allow individuals to commit to new behaviors. Once they understand the relevance of new information and its potential influence on areas they are interested in, then they can consider various options and appreciate the importance of altering their current behavior.

The most challenging aspect of my personal attempts to influence physician behavior is an inability to bring the individuals around the table to have the conversation in the first place. It appears that they are too engaged in the present way of responding to find the time to discover new and potentially better solutions. Seemingly, persisting and complaining are easier than allocating the time to discover creative, new responses.

According to Chuck Dwyer (1992), you can make people an offer they cannot refuse if you change their perception that engaging in the behavior *you* seek will serve to enhance what *they* personally value.

A person's behavior makes perfectly good sense from her point of view. To get her to willingly commit to new behaviors requires changing that point of view. A person's behavior is in service of her personal hierarchy of needs or values. Whether I choose to attend my son's soccer game or to stay late at the office is a reflection of my personal hierarchy of needs/values. What I value is important, but the order in which I value them is even more important. When I cannot have them both—when I must choose—I will choose the one that is more important.

While my behavior is in service of my personal hierarchy of needs/values, the choice of specific behaviors is guided by my existing operating assumptions, beliefs, and attitudes. Members of street gangs behave differently from people in mainstream society. You might be tempted to conclude that their needs/values must be different. However, if you talk to a gang member and ask why he behaves the way he does, he will frequently respond that the gang is his family, the gang trusts and respects each other, and the other members love him like a brother. Family, trust, respect, and love are highly ordered values within mainstream society as well. Gang members behave differently because they believe that those values are enhanced by behaving according to the norms of the gang. The same values are enhanced for mainstream citizens by behaving according to the socialized norms of their peer group. The choice of specific behaviors, then, is guided by existing beliefs and operating assumptions.

To make someone an offer he cannot refuse, you must know what he values. Many individuals, and this is especially true of physician scientists, have never explicitly identified what they value or how they rank order their values. Without being consciously aware of what you value, you cannot knowingly make choices in service of those values. If choices are made without consideration of your personal values hierarchy, you can be unaware of your own contribution to creating a sense of dissatisfaction with present circumstances. Helping individuals identify and prioritize what they value most is a very useful way to begin to build partnership.

In order for someone to willingly commit to new behaviors, she must change her existing operating assumptions, beliefs, or attitudes. This is only possible by presenting to that individual data that addresses the level of belief that sustains the current way of behaving. As stated previously, this dynamic is facilitated through dialogue. Essentially, you allow someone to conclude for himself that changing his behavior better serves his self-interest.

This process is like redecorating a room. The possibilities of what you might select to put *in* the room have no end. The challenge is deciding what you are willing to take *out* of the room. Metaphorically speaking, the pieces of furniture you remove are the operating assumptions and existing beliefs that you are now willing to dismiss as invalid. Creativity is intertwined with destruction. To willingly commit to new behaviors, existing assumptions, beliefs, or attitudes need to be destroyed.

An overwhelming number of physicians value respect, control, fair reimbursement, efficiency, improvements in patient care, and time. If you can allow physicians to see that engaging in the behavior you seek, rather than their current behavior, will serve to better enhance one of these values, they might change that behavior. Remember, however, that the hierarchy of needs/values is of pivotal importance. If control is valued more than time, and what you propose delivering is incremental time at the expense of control, then your offer may well be refused.

Understanding the motivational sequence is important. When you seek to make an offer that cannot be refused, you are offering a quid pro quo. If the person changes her way of behaving, she will get more of something that she values. The motivational sequence involves three specific questions (Elkind 2004):

1. Is what you propose possible? If the answer to this question is no, there is no deal. You must be able to make your case that what you promise will indeed accrue as a result of new behavior.
2. Are you capable? The answer to this question should be rated low, medium, or high. Your challenge is to move the answer toward the high end of the spectrum. Fundamentally, you ask the question, "What would it take to allow you to feel that you are highly capable of this new behavior?" Then, you must provide this resource.
3. Is it worthwhile—that is, do you want to? This question is really the only important one. Again, the answer to this question should be rated low, medium, or high, and your challenge is to move it toward the high end of the spectrum. If the individual does not strongly want to engage in this behavior, then it tends to go to the bottom of his to-do list, where it becomes rather improbable.

KNOW THE PLAYERS

Everett Rogers (1995), Tom Atchison (2005), Malcolm Gladwell (2000), and Manny Elkind (2004) have presented constructs that allow for identifying segments within a community that have the capacity to more rapidly promote and disseminate change. Those who are attempting to influence physician behavior should become familiar with Rogers's (1995) observations on the dissemination of innovation. Some physicians are disproportionately effective at influencing the general physician community. With respect to a willingness to change behavior, Rogers segments any community into five distinct groups:

1. Innovators
2. Early adopters
3. Early majority
4. Late majority
5. Laggards

Innovators comprise between 2 and 3 percent of any community. They actively seek new ideas and tend to dance at the fringes of everyone's paradigm. Their primary contribution to the community at large is to be magnets for new ideas. All new ideas are imported. Innovators scan the horizon and identify new possibilities. However, innovators have very little influence on the rest of the community. Because they constantly flitter from one new idea to another, others in the community cannot ascertain whether they are genius or crazy.

Early adopters are like innovators in that they see possibilities in novelty. Unlike innovators, they are influential in the community at large and often serve as the opinion leaders for the group. They take new ideas and "reinvent them locally." They adapt the ideas to the local circumstances, taking into account local resources, history, and other relevant factors.

Unlike the innovators and early adopters, who are open to new ideas, the rest of the community takes no cues from outside and are focused internally. The *early majority* are influenced by the behavior of the early adopters. When the early majority see the early adopters successfully adapting new behaviors, they will begin to copy that behavior. Once this occurs, innovation cannot be stopped.

The *late majority* is even slower to adopt new behaviors, and *laggards* often refuse to participate. Laggards, however, should not be dismissed. They often represent connections to the meaningful past. Many times, they offer reflections that bridge to the historical purpose of the group and prevent the group from abandoning traditions of importance.

The innovators and early adopters, who together comprise approximately 15 percent of any group and who, according to Rogers, are open to the importation of new ideas, are distinguished from the remainder of the group by their willingness to risk. The others are risk averse. Given constraints on time and monetary resources, it would behoove those seeking to influence physician behavior to focus their efforts on the early adopters.

In an analogous fashion, Tom Atchison (2005) has categorized the physician community into five distinct groups:

1. Proactive leaders
2. Reactive followers
3. Uncertains
4. Skeptics
5. Cynics

Proactive leaders are similar to Rogers's innovators and early adopters. *Reactive followers* are like the early majority; they can be influenced to adopt new behaviors, but they do not want to go first.

Atchison's characterization of the uncertains, skeptics, and cynics adds additional understanding. *Uncertains*, as the title implies, are individuals who can side either with those who are willing to adopt new behaviors and align with the healthcare organization, or with those who defend the historical status quo. If organizational leaders pay a disproportionate amount of attention to those who seek to maintain the status quo rather than nurture the more progressive and aligned members of the medical community, the uncertains may conclude that their individual needs can be met better by complaining than by complying. Many healthcare organization leaders spend a disproportionate amount of time trying to convince resistors, especially if they are "big admitters," rather than promoting those who share the organizational vision. In doing this, they risk shifting the uncertains and losing the support of this middle-of-the-road group.

Cynics, who comprise approximately 1 to 3 percent of the group, never offer a positive contribution. They seek to enhance their own stature by being critical of others. These constant complainers disproportionately occupy the time of hospital administrators. They never add anything constructive to the dialogue. Atchison advises that either you ignore them or confront them to identify the specifics of their negatively critical attack, state that they never seem to have anything positive to contribute, and challenge them to present a better idea. Most of the time, the cynics will retreat. If, by some miracle, they actually present a positive idea, publicly put them in charge of implementing that idea.

Do not to misidentify skeptics as cynics. *Skeptics* make positive contributions by pointing out the negative. Skeptics are very critical thinkers and are quick to identify defects or inadequacies in proposed initiatives. Because the nature of their response is primarily identifying the negatives, too often the skeptic is seen as being unsupportive or as a detractor, rather than as a potentially supportive constructive critic.

If you can pay attention to skeptics' criticisms and modify your proposal in accordance with their recommendations, they often will move from being a skeptic to being a proactive leader on this specific initiative. Atchison points out that an accrual of support does not exist among skeptics. You must win them over each time you seek to involve them in an initiative.

Early adopters, proactive leaders, and potentially skeptics catalyze change.

Another useful way of segmenting the medical community to maximize your ability to influence physician behavior is described by Malcolm Gladwell (2000). The following list identifies Gladwell's three types of disproportionately influential individuals who catalyze ideas through a community:

1. *Connectors* are the equivalent of a human Rolodex. They are rapid disseminators of information. They seem to move in a variety of circles and serve to transfer information over a wide area.
2. *Mavens* are individuals who seem to know something about everything and who delight in sharing that information with no personal gain. Because they are not self-serving, others trust them.
3. *Salesmen* have the capacity to tap into and influence the emotional state of other people around them. This group is disproportionately influential.

I strongly recommend reading Gladwell's book, *The Tipping Point*, in which he describes the adoption of new behaviors as metaphorically analogous to the spread of epidemics. The analogy is quite strong, and the lessons are readily adaptable to initiatives aimed at influencing physician behavior. If you can identify those members of your medical community who serve as connectors, mavens, or especially salesmen, you can more effectively disseminate and promote supportive new ideas and behaviors.

Manny Elkind (2004) teaches a useful distinction. People segregate into groups labeled matchers and mismatchers. Individuals seem to have a propensity to see in either similarity or dissimilarity. *Matchers* are quite comfortable focusing on similarity. *Mismatchers*, on the other hand, have a predilection for focusing on dissimilarity. In the earlier context, skeptics are mismatchers. They primarily focus on dissimilarity. Internists are often mismatchers because they are taught to think in terms of "rule-outs." Mismatchers make positive contributions by identifying the negatives in any proposal. They are often mislabeled as naysayers, saboteurs, or nonsupporters, when in fact they see their critical remarks as positive contributions to the final product. When engaging a mismatcher, assess their overall response to the proposal that is being presented by asking, "On a scale of 1 to 10 how do you find this proposal?" In this way, you can get an overview of their impressions and avoid quickly assuming that they reject the idea out of hand because their first comments are negative.

LEAD TO CRITICAL MASS

All groups act to defend the status quo. According to Rogers (1995), only 15 percent of any group (innovators and early adopters) can imagine possibilities in novelty and are willing to consider adopting a new paradigm. Since in a town-hall democracy a majority of the group must vote in favor of a proposal for it to be adopted, physicians collectively reject all truly new ideas. Therefore, to promote change, you must be willing to lead not to consensus, but rather to critical mass. Critical mass has been empirically defined as the square root of n. Change nothing, but pilot everything!

I would like to introduce the idea of approaching change using the metaphor of moving a slinky. The early adopters represent the front rings of the slinky, the square root of n. Pilot new ideas with the early adopters. The success of those ideas is analogous to pulling the front rings away from the other rings, creating a tension that will cause the remaining rings of the slinky to seek to catch up with the front rings in their own time.

Managing to consensus would be analogous to trying to push the slinky from behind thereby having to overcome the inertia of the entire group.

APPRECIATE DIVERSITY

Appreciate that excellence is a form of deviant behavior. You become excellent because you are doing things that "normal" people do not want to do. This represents a statistical truism. For any observation to be seen as different from others, it must exist outside of two standard deviations of the mean of the population of observations in question. Distinctively exceptional behavior, therefore, represents deviancy. This concept is synchronous with the notion of piloting new behaviors with early adopters, who are seeking to achieve superior results through innovative, creative approaches.

Another approach differs from the usual attempts to change physician behavior. People have a natural tendency to focus on what is wrong or missing. Through identifying the negative, we seek to transform it or replace it with something that, we hope, will be a more successful behavior. Seeking to achieve change through appreciative inquiry takes a converse approach (Cooperrider and Witney 2005). Rather than focusing on what is missing, appreciative inquiry seeks to identify elements of the desired behavior already in evidence. After analyzing why or how those desired elements are already present, those wanting to create the change import and replicate those critical elements into other areas within the organization.

By understanding the factors that allow for the expression of this behavior in those settings, you can promote its expression in others. By showing that the desired behavior already exists, you can emphasize that segments within the organization are already successfully practicing the new behavior. This promotes a can-do attitude. Others within the organization can readily appreciate that success is possible, because success is already present somewhere else in the organization. Moreover, that it is already present locally creates legitimacy in the minds of the risk-averse 85 percent of the population who only accept cues from inside (Rogers 1995).

One aspect of appreciative inquiry is the concept of positive deviancy (Sternin 2003). The few individuals within an organization who already manifest the desired behavior become the focal point of investigation—the positive deviants. Again, this approach studies what allows the few individuals who already behave as desired to stand out as exceptions rather than focus on those who fail to manifest the desired behavior. By identifying what promotes the successful manifestation of the desired behavior, those variables can be shared in a way that promotes the behavior in the rest of the group. For this to work, the positive deviants must be subject to the same constraints as everyone else in the group; the larger group must be allowed to repetitively practice the new behavior; and there must be in place a metric that provides positive feedback that reinforces the new behavior.

PUT IT TOGETHER

Identify Shared Interests

In seeking to influence physician behavior, start at points of agreement. If the interests of individual stakeholders are represented as circles, areas of shared interest and/or agreement are shown where the circles overlap. Initiatives that address the aligned areas of self-interest are desired by everyone and would achieve collective support. This seems to be a simple concept, yet, in my experience, rather than seeking to identify areas of shared and common interest, conversations almost invariably degenerate into arguments over which position is more correct.

Focus on the Future

In addition to focusing on areas of agreement, remain focused on the future. Focusing on the future creates hope, whereas focusing on the past degenerates into arguments over who is to blame for the current state of affairs. For the same reason, begin from where things are, not from where they ought to be. I am amazed at the amount of time that is wasted talking about how things should be rather than accepting them as they are. Wishing that things were different is not an effective strategy.

Remove Barriers

Remove barriers whenever possible. When you can remove an existing barrier, you become an instant hero. You do not have to convince anyone of the value achieved by taking away a known negative. Doing so achieves instant credibility and builds trust. Physicians usually appreciate making processes more efficient, thereby saving time and reducing frustration (especially when they do not have to modify their own behavior in the process).

By contrast, attempts to introduce a new and hopefully positive change are far more likely to generate skepticism. Moreover, the adoption of new behaviors is not always met by the hoped-for positive results. This journey into the unknown is often more cautious and less enthusiastic, and failure erodes confidence and trust. For example, physicians have resisted many of the initiatives aimed at enhancing patient safety. They are often reluctant to participate in electronic physician order entry or medication verification, and these initiatives have not resulted in the anticipated benefits.

Remember Columbo and the Veg-O-Matic Salesman

My two favorite role models for influencing physician behavior are Columbo and the Veg-O-Matic salesman, Ron Popeil. Columbo appears as a naïve novice, deferential to the suspect in question. He plants ideas in the form of questions and cautious hypotheses. By analogy, make new ideas appear to be owned by those whose behavior you seek to influence. Planting seeds through Socratic questioning is a very effective approach. No one likes to be told what to do.

The Veg-O-Matic salesman is successful because he never appears to be selling. His approach is to first identify with the frustrations that are experienced by those he seeks to influence. By identifying with their frustrations, he gains acceptance. They appreciate that he understands their circumstances. After identifying with their frustrations, he asks if they would be interested in resolving those frustrations. He then introduces the potential solution to their problems, and, at that point, they are eager to buy.

In a similar way, it is important to appreciate the points of frustration that annoy physicians. In many ways, seek to be a servant leader, one who understands and empathizes with the perspectives and needs of others. By trying to resolve their needs, you gain acceptance, credibility, and trust.

Too often, we approach physicians because we see them as important to achieving our objectives. We are perceived as selling, and they become guarded and resistant. If we can begin by identifying with their frustrations and allowing them to see that our proposal holds the promise of ameliorating those frustrations, physicians can become eager buyers and willing participants.

Resolve the "Yeah, But..." Response

In seeking to promote new behaviors, a useful approach involves attempting to resolve the "Yeah, but…" response that invariably surfaces (Morgan 1997). Individuals can appreciate the potential value that attends your proposal. As they listen to your proposal, they respond with a series of "Yeahs" as they appreciate the potential positives in what you propose.

At the conclusion of your presentation, however, they are quick to say, "But…." The "but" identifies elements in their current behavior that they believe produce deliverables that are important to them. So, while they see the potential in your proposal, they fear loss of the deliverables that accompany their current way of behaving. Seeking to resolve this tension allows you to identify middle ground. Seek to introduce the new while preserving the critical elements of the old.

Ask the Right Type of Questions

I would like to caution you against conducting physician focus groups or asking individual physicians to respond to your ideas by asking, "What do you think?" Several potentially negative consequences result:

- If the physician likes what you are proposing, he will likely hold you responsible for creating the result. Asking the question creates an expectation.
- The response to your idea will end up being the sum and substance of the physician's contribution to achieving the result. Giving the advice would be the equivalent of serving as the architect on the project.

It is far better to approach the physician or physicians by asking, "If this is a good idea, what could we do together to bring it about?" Framing the question in this way achieves two important outcomes. The physician's response will be much more measured, and, when the time comes to initiate the project, you can seek to engage her in the activities that she identified. What you want is not only input, but also engagement.

Use Dialogue to Reach Collective Wisdom

I would again like to emphasize the critical importance of dialogue. Nothing meaningful happens outside of conversation. The answers to all problems are in the collective wisdom of the assembled group. As Margaret Wheatley (1994) said, "When people of shared purpose are given access to the relevant data and allowed to engage in soulful dialogue, magic happens."

SUMMARY

A successful pathway to influencing physicians involves the following:

- Develop trust. Remember that you build trust not only through transformational relationships that express vulnerability, but also through a willingness to understand physician needs and perspectives.

- Engage physicians in Socratic dialogue, allowing them to make sense of your proposal, connect the dots for themselves, and create meaning.
- Appreciate that all behavior is in service of an individual's hierarchy of needs and that the choice of specific behavior rests on existing beliefs and operating assumptions. Getting others to commit to new behaviors requires changing their perception to believe that engaging in the behavior you seek will serve to enhance what they value.
- Create change as you would move a slinky, focusing on the disproportionately influential early adopters, proactive leaders, and converted skeptics.
- Focus on success by utilizing appreciative inquiry, starting from where things are and not from where they ought to be. Emphasize points of agreement.
- Remove barriers.

Also, understand the importance of positive vision. A negative vision seeks to make something go away. The intensity of the negative stimulus will cause people to commit to action. While negative vision can galvanize people to act, it never sustains change. In essence, the intensity of the need to respond generates the response. The response reduces the intensity of the stimulus, simultaneously reducing the motivation to act. The result is a saw-tooth pattern of activity. Positive vision, on the other hand, seeks to bring something new into being. People embrace a vision not for what it says but for what it does, not because it is probable, but rather because it is irresistible. Positive visions are sustaining. Articulating that positive vision is the primary responsibility of leadership.

NOTE

1. Quoted in Mardy Grothe, *Oxymoronica: Paradoxical Wit and Wisdom from History's Greatest Wordsmiths* (New York: HarperCollins, 2004), 91.

REFERENCES

Atchison, T. 2005. Personal communication with the author.

Cooperrider, D. L., and D. L. Witney. 2005. *Collaborating for Change: Appreciative Inquiry*. San Francisco: Berrett-Koehler.

Dwyer, C. E. 1992. *The Shifting Sources of Power and Influence*. Tampa, FL: American College of Physician Executives.

Elkind, M. 2004. Personal communication with the author.

Gladwell, M. 2000. *The Tipping Point*. Boston: Little Brown.

Lencioni, P. 2002. *The Five Dysfunctions of a Team*. San Francisco: Jossey Bass.

Morgan, G. 1997. *Images of Organization*, 2nd ed. Thousand Oaks, CA: Sage Publications.

Rogers, E. M. 1995. *Diffusions of Innovations*. New York: Free Press.

Shaw, P. 2002. *Changing Conversations in Organizations*. London: Routledge.

Sternin, J. 2003. "Practice Positive Deviance for Extraordinary Social and Change." In *The Change Champion's Field Guide: Strategies and Tools for Leading Change in Your Organization*, edited by D. Ulrich, M. Goldsmith, L. Carter, J. Bolt, and N. Smallwood. Boston: Best Practice Publications, 20–37.

Wheatley, M. 1994. *Leadership and the New Science Revised: Discovering Order in a Chaotic World*. San Francisco: Berrett-Koehler.

CHAPTER 4

Structural Changes that Can Align Physicians with Healthcare Organizations

It's tough to make predictions, especially about the future.
—Yogi Berra[1]

THREE APPROACHES TO PHYSICIAN RELATIONSHIPS

Healthcare organizations are dependent on physicians to care for patients. Because of the forces that are affecting the provider community, relationships between healthcare organizations and physicians are becoming more complex. Healthcare organizations must develop a strategic approach to physician relationships. It seems clear to me that the traditional medical staff organization is not the way to develop relationships with physicians. A robust pluralistic approach is necessary.

In essence, healthcare organizations can approach physician relationships in three ways. First, they can choose to court physicians. All physicians appreciate changes that produce improvements in patient care and that simplify and streamline patient-care processes. A physician is more likely to be attracted to caring for patients in a healthcare-organization setting if his workday is made easier. Since improvements in patient outcomes and reduction in the cost of care usually accompany enhanced efficiency, this approach is a win-win for both parties. Facilitating operating room throughput would be one good example. Starting the first case on time, shortening time between cases, having all the necessary information available for the scheduled pre-incision "huddle," and operating with the same personnel would be very attractive to any surgeon and create strong loyalties in the process.

Second, some healthcare organizations have chosen to directly compete with members of their physician community. When physicians choose to care for patients in their own facilities, these healthcare organizations recruit similar specialists to work within the organization. Some organizations have gone so far as to deny hospital privileges to members of the physician community who have chosen to directly compete with the hospital. In this approach, physicians are categorized as being either with the healthcare organization or against it. Other organizations have taken a less absolute position and chosen to exclude competing physicians from positions of strategic or tactical importance, such as chief of staff or head of departments, or from important medical staff committees.

The third approach is to collaborate with physicians. This approach seeks to create economic win-win initiatives. When faced with the choice of either competing with the physicians or collaborating with them, these healthcare organizations decide "one half a loaf is better than none." More to the point, the most successful healthcare organizations move beyond a reluctant, passive approach to physician partnership and seek to create a synergistic, non–zero-sum game relationship that benefits both parties.

Physician Employment

Many physicians are seeking employment. Most Generation X physicians expect it. Growing regulatory and payer demands, shrinking physician profit margins, educational debt, and generational attitudes that dominantly value a balanced life come together to promote health-care organizations employing physicians. Historically, healthcare organizations have sought to employ primary care physicians as a way of funneling patients to specialty physicians who are aligned with the hospital. Now, employing the specialists themselves is a growing trend, as evidenced by the expanding presence of employed intensivists, hospitalists, trauma surgeons, and physicians who are hired to serve as service-line medical directors. This phenomonon is further evidenced by preferred contractual relationships with pathologists, anesthesiologists, emergency department physicians, and radiologists as sole providers of their respective services.

The accelerating trend of paying physicians to take emergency department calls is prompting some hospitals to hire physicians who are employed specifically to meet this responsibility. The total cost of paying everyone to take calls often equals or exceeds that of specif-ically employing a small number of individuals.

For example, in many communities, orthopedic surgeons are refusing to take emergency calls unless hospitals pay them an amount that never seems to remain satisfactory. Often, it starts as a stipend per day of call. Then, the expectation accelerates to an additional subsidy for caring for patients who lack health insurance or who are covered by agencies that reimburse at less than the amount paid by the best payer source. The number of days in a month times the cost per day soon totals a sum that equals the yearly salaries plus benefits required to employ three orthopedic surgeons who would take calls as part of their employed relation-ship. The revenues generated by the surgical procedures that fol-low caring for patients with orthopedic emergencies can often off-set the costs of the program.

When healthcare organizations can specifically contract with or employ fewer physicians to provide care, they can build into the rela-tionships defined expectations for performance. These expectations can create predictability and quality of performance in the processes and outcomes of care. This is far easier to achieve than working with a larger number of unaligned physicians on a voluntary medical staff.

The growing shortage of certain medical specialists like intensivists, hospitalists, and neurosurgeons complicates these initiatives. Demand exceeds supply. Competition to hire those specialists is significantly driving up the cost of physician employment.

Expanding Scope of Medical Staff Services

Many healthcare organizations are expanding departments devoted to physician relationships. Primary care physicians are removing themselves from the hospital setting. Multiple factors are responsible:

- The growing complexity of healthcare
- Credentialing and privileging criteria that marginalize primary care physicians, especially in more urban settings
- A reimbursement system that is biased against cognitive specialties and fails to economically reward relationship-based specialties
- The increasing cost of malpractice insurance
- The economic reality that a primary care physician can earn more income at less personal cost by seeing patients in her office than by driving to and from multiple hospitals

Generation X attitudes that primarily value a balanced life further reinforce physicians' desire to limit patient care responsibilities to defined and controlled hours.

Because healthcare organizations significantly benefit from the referrals that are directed by primary care physicians, they should maintain a close relationship with and promote the loyalty of their primary care community. Healthcare organizations seek to nurture this relationship by linking physicians to the healthcare organization through information systems, reduced overhead because of group purchasing arrangements, and "back office" management initiatives. In addition, healthcare organizations seek to streamline the ability to provide diagnostic services with short turnaround times for their patients. A close working relationship with hospitalists, in which the primary care physician is kept thoroughly informed regarding the status of his hospitalized patients, is very important.

Traditionally, the office of medical staff affairs existed to respond to physician complaints, support credentialing and privileging, and facilitate continuing medical education. This presented a reactive position that was intended to put out fires or smooth ruffled feathers. Progressive departments now proactively facilitate the physician's ability to remain compliant with expanding regulatory requirements. The most sophisticated departments act strategically to anticipate and position the provider community for success by assessing emerging physician needs, technology trends, and changing patient and payer expectations. These are ways that promote healthcare organization–physician relationships along a continuum that can extend from mutual appreciation through degrees of economic partnerships that include service-line direction, co-management, joint ventures, and employment. An attitude that seeks to first identify with the physician's needs and then seeks to facilitate their success is the foundation for creating and maintaining a trusting and loyal relationship. Unfortunately, the doctor is too often viewed as someone who must be leveraged to serve the organization's needs. That approach only serves to promote suspicion and erodes the trust essential for enduring and successful relationships.

As relationships between healthcare organizations and physicians continue to evolve, and as physician workforce shortages become more acute, some medical staff offices have begun to employ physician recruiters. This is an attempt to proactively position the healthcare organization for success in this highly competitive endeavor.

Collaborative Mindset

Healthcare organizations seeking to collaborate with members of their physician community need to define the shared purpose and the shared values that will accompany the relationship. The organization must explicitly define what the relationship's purpose is, the compelling rationale behind the relationship, the value hierarchy that will guide decision making, and the metrics that will be applied to define success.

Remember that physicians, as members of an expert culture, are motivated primarily by vision and not mission. When the organization's goals align with individual physician self-interest, success will follow. In addition, since the business plan must serve the organization's purpose, physician participants must be educated in the economics that accompany the shared enterprise. Marketplace dynamics are not part of the medical curriculum, and most physicians would benefit from a crash course in medical economics. Because of the growing trend toward consumerism in healthcare, a critical element for success is the transition from focusing on the *provider* to focusing on the *customer*.

Ambulatory care is contributing progressively more revenue to healthcare organizations. Because the core competencies of hospitals are directed at acute care intervention, most healthcare organizations are ill prepared to efficiently manage ambulatory-based services. If ambulatory-based services are run with the same mindset that manages the departmentalized budgeting process driving most healthcare organizations, the enterprise will fail.

CHALLENGES

Two great challenges confront today's healthcare organization. The first is deciding if the organization should "stick to its knitting" and remain focused on delivering acute care, or expand beyond the traditional and move into diagnostic, preventive, and ambulatory-based interventional services. Even more challenging is whether the healthcare organization should move beyond delivering wholesale services toward providing retail services as well. The whole range of complementary and alternative medical interventions and the provision of services not currently reimbursed through third-party payers represent expanding markets that are not traditionally served by allopathic medicine.

The second major challenge is simultaneously specializing and integrating. The growing trend toward progressive specialization, with its focused-factory approach, presents a dilemma. The narrow focus creates enhanced efficiency and effectiveness of the services rendered. However, it simultaneously isolates and fragments care. The growing presence of physician extenders, who provide a limited range of services in commercial establishments such as Wal-Mart and drugstores, together with urgent care centers and services provided via the Internet, also contribute.

Clinic Model

If the provision of high quality and safe patient care is dependent on the integration of patient care information, how is this to be accomplished in light of the growing fragmentation of healthcare services?

Perhaps the clinic model represents the best solution. The trends toward employing physician specialists and developing a complete electronic medical record are driving a more complete and inclusive relationship between the traditional healthcare organization and selected members of the physician community. The Mayo Clinic, Cleveland Clinic, Kaiser-Permanente, Veterans Health Administration, and multispecialty physician-group practices that take over and manage hospitals (e.g., Billings Clinic and the Carilion Clinic) are some examples.

Optimal Reimbursement

Perhaps the next generation of pay-for-performance initiatives that seek to provide a fair reimbursement for an expanded range of services that are integrated across multiple specialties will represent an economic force that promotes the integration of care. These initiatives would seek to define episodes of care and/or disease management approaches as packaged services that are accountable for the quality of the outcomes created in return for fair reimbursement.

ADAPTABILITY

Given that change is progressing exponentially and that the future is unknowable, perhaps a complexity lens provides the most useful metaphor for guiding relationships (Zimmerman 1998). Adaptability is the key to sustainability. Healthcare is a complex adaptive system, a densely connected web of interacting agents, each operating from its own schema or local knowledge.

For example, physicians, nurses, hospitals, payers, regulators, the technology industry, the pharmaceutical industry, and other agencies play together in the healthcare sandbox. Each agent makes decisions in response to changes that are occurring within the industry in an attempt to maximize its own interests. The consequences (output) of the decisions made by one agent become the input that prompts a reactive response from the other agents that are affected by those decisions. In a nonlinear fashion, the entire system progressively evolves to adapt to an increasingly complex external environment.

Agents co-evolve with the complex adaptive system of which they are a part. The cause and effect is mutual rather than one-way. The system is emerging from a dense pattern of interactions. Complex adaptive systems have the following attributes:

- They are nonlinear.
- They learn from experience and can therefore modify their response to a given stimulus.
- They are history dependent.

In being history dependent, the nature of the response is influenced by historical preconditions. That is, the consequences of a given response to change can be uniquely different. Universal laws do not bring all developments to the same predetermined endpoint. Attempts to impose templates on unique organizations will fail unless sensitive to and adapted to unique pre-existing conditions.

Within complex adaptive systems, diversity enhances the potential for success. Diverse elements have to be connected to maximize the potential that is inherent in a multiplicity of viewpoints. For the organization to be maximally adaptive, there also needs to be distributed control. That is, the best outcomes emerge when an entity organizes itself, rather than having an organization imposed by the top of a command-and-control structure.

Leadership and Adaptability

In the complexity metaphor, leadership is about managing context and relationships. Leaders need to think less like managers and more like gardeners. Gardeners do not grow crops; they create conditions in which crops grow (Morgan 1997). Leaders establish the boundaries of the enterprise and identify the minimum specifications that must be incorporated into solutions. Then, they provide the necessary information to people of shared purpose and allow them to engage in meaningful dialogue (Wheatley 2004). Then, magic happens. In essence, a sense of shared purpose and shared values creates a container within which individuals self-organize and, through dialogue, find creative solutions.

This certainly represents a departure from the current way healthcare organizations are structured. Healthcare organizations continue to reflect an industrial model of top-down hierarchical structure. It is imperative that relationships be founded on explicitly defined shared purpose and shared values. This provides the glue that facilitates adaptive response to a rapidly changing and challenging healthcare environment.

SUMMARY

Advancing technology and economic pressures are positioning physicians as the dominant competitor to healthcare organizations. The historical ways of relating are no longer applicable. No longer can the healthcare organization view itself as the physician's workshop, with a need to treat all doctors equally. The healthcare organization must decide how it is to relate to the physician community. Will it court them, committing to simplifying processes and to becoming more efficient as ways to increase physicians' convenience and, thus, their loyalty? Will it directly compete? Or, will it choose to collaborate? In any case, new structures and new processes will need to be designed to accommodate new relationships. Currently, there is momentum toward employing physicians as a way of aligning incentives and placing doctors in positions of management. Other forces are challenging healthcare organizations to move into the ambulatory sector to compete for discretionary dollars.

The rapid pace of change limits the duration of effectiveness of business models and demands that relationships be founded on shared purpose and values. In such a world, a complexity science metaphor provides a more useful approach than the traditional top-down, command-and-control model better suited for times of stability.

NOTE

1. Quoted in Mardy Grothe, *Oxymoronica: Paradoxical Wit and Wisdom from History's Greatest Wordsmiths* (New York: HarperCollins, 2004), 220.

REFERENCES

Morgan, G. 1997. *Images of Organization*. Thousand Oaks, CA: Sage Publications.

Wheatley, M. 1994. *Leadership and the New Science Revised: Discovering Order in a Chaotic World*. San Francisco: Berrett-Koehler.

Zimmerman, B. 1998. *Edgeware*. Irving, TX: VHA.

CHAPTER 5

Why Physicians Are Barriers to Achieving Improvements in Patient Safety and Clinical Quality

It infuriates me to be wrong when I know I'm right.

—Molière[1]

DEMANDS TO IMPROVE PATIENT SAFETY AND CLINICAL QUALITY

There are three important drivers for hospitals to improve patient safety and clinical quality. The first are professional and moral obligations to do so. Providers of healthcare services should intrinsically desire to maximize the outcomes of their interventions. The second is a strong business case that supports improvement initiatives. The elimination of unnecessary interventions and the avoidance of costly adverse effects have positive economic consequences when reimbursement is fixed and predetermined, as is the case with Medicare and Medicaid. The third is an increasing number of regulatory requirements that expect compliance with identified processes of care that contribute to enhancements in patient safety and the quality of clinical outcomes.

Significant Geographical Variation

Subsequent to the publishing of the *Dartmouth Atlas*, demands have grown for public reporting of data that will allow payers and patients to better judge the value received for their healthcare dollar. The *Dartmouth Atlas* has documented the wide geographical variation with which patient care interventions are applied. With many different approaches to the same diagnosis, which one is the better? How do patients determine if they are undergoing unnecessary interventions, or if necessary interventions are being withheld?

Similarly, payers and patients may naturally question why, if strong medical evidence supports given interventions, those specific interventions are not applied 100 percent of the time when that given condition is present. Allopathic medicine prides itself on being scientifically based. The prospective, double-blind, randomized trial, with a significant number of participants and a demonstrated P value greater than .05, is the gold standard. However, the frequency with which evidence-based interventions are actually applied widely varies. This has led to demands for the public reporting of data in attempts to drive initiatives that seek to achieve the appropriate application of these interventions 100 percent of the time when indicated.

Hospitalized Patients Are at Risk

Subsequent to the 1999 publishing of the first Institute of Medicine report, *To Err Is Human*, in which it was estimated that as many as 98,000 individuals per year die because of hospitalization, there has been a growing demand that hospitals engineer environments that protect patients from untoward events.

Payers Are Demanding Changes

Payers are attempting to drive changes within the provider community. The Leapfrog Group was the first high-profile association that sought to influence the structure and processes of care in support of changes that could ensure higher quality and safer patient care. The Leapfrog Group focused on the value of utilizing intensivist physicians, the relationship between volume and outcome, and the enhancements in patient safety that accompany physician electronic order entry. Each of these significantly increases the quality of medical outcome and reduces patient risk. The businesses that composed the Leapfrog Group would direct their employees to preferentially seek treatment at healthcare organizations that could meet those standards of care. Similarly, pay-for-performance initiatives seek to couple incremental payment to the demonstrated application of evidence-based interventions. Conversely, payers are beginning to deny payment for preventable complications that affect hospitalized patients.

Reducing Variation Improves Clinical Outcome

Payers, regulators, and providers of healthcare services are focusing on standardizing processes of care in attempts to reduce variation. These initiatives are rooted in total quality management as currently embodied in Toyota Lean Production and Six Sigma. These approaches seek to eliminate waste and achieve perfection. Reducing variation is seen as a way of enhancing efficiency and improving the effectiveness of healthcare, and standardization of processes helps to ensure patient safety. Historically, the medical community has confined its quality-focused efforts, such as they exist, around quality assurance in support of physician credentialing and privileging. These efforts originated with a focus on risk management that seeks to identify practitioners who represented a threat to patients, and thereby to the organization's reputation and malpractice exposure. This then expanded to a focus on quality assurance, wherein clinicians were expected to achieve minimum standards of performance when caring for patients. Quality assurance activities render judgments about appropriate training, skill development, and demonstrated competency, and they are necessarily individual-practitioner–focused and retrospective.

Healthcare Emphasizes Personal Accountability

Healthcare is a culture of personal accountability. Quality assurance initiatives begin from an adverse outcome. A retrospective analysis of the care provided follows. In these circumstances you can always identify more than one individual who, if only they had been paying attention, could have prevented the adverse outcome from occurring. Once the individuals involved have been identified, a demand for additional training is made in the hopes that their skill level, competency, or knowledge deficiency will be enhanced or corrected. Healthcare providers are not taught to think in terms of processes of care. Rather, individual competency is the focus, and healthcare providers rely on vigilance and memory to avoid mistakes and maximize outcomes of care.

Nothing can happen to a patient in the absence of a physician order. Primary accountability, therefore, rests with the physician who writes the order. America's tort system further reinforces individual accountability. Professional training, the provider culture, and legal and historical imperatives all directly conflict with approaches that emphasize the standardization of processes of care.

Other Cultural Barriers

Two additional cultural elements interfere with the safety and quality agenda. The first is a belief that *knowing* equals *doing*. It is as if the only tool in the provider-community toolbox useful for driving the safety and quality agenda is the sharing of information. Knowledge is a necessary precondition to change, but it is far from sufficient. Yet, in a culture in which individual autonomy is prized above every other value, it is assumed that good people who are given access to good information will make correct decisions and adjust their behavior accordingly. Knowledge is not enough; capacity and motivation are also necessary. The most important attribute to the change process is wanting to change.

The other cultural norm is related to the concept of "no harm, no foul." When adverse medical events are studied, traditionally they are graded on a continuum from one to five. At level one, nothing adverse occurred. At level five, the patient died. Traditional quality assurance approaches typically do not assess adverse outcomes unless the result is at least at a level three. This often violates the principle of the inverse power law. The inverse power law is a relationship that points to a common cause for effects of a varying magnitude. When the frequency of the outcome squared plotted against the magnitude of the outcome squared results in a downward sloping straight line, it indicates an identical causal mechanism (Poole et al. 2000). For example, the most common consequence of a patient with a stated history of penicillin allergy inadvertently receiving penicillin is that nothing adverse occurs (i.e., the outcome with the highest frequency occurs at the lowest magnitude). Once every several years, a patient may die from an anaphylactic response (i.e., the response of the greatest magnitude occurs with the lowest frequency). In both instances, the process failure that resulted in the patient receiving penicillin in the first place may be identical. However, in the healthcare community, the event is rarely investigated when nothing adverse occurs.

Quality Improvement Focuses on Process

In contrast to quality assurance, quality improvement initiatives are prospective and process focused. They attempt to improve the aggregate outcome of care for all patients with a given condition. Quality improvement initiatives seek to identify those interventions and processes that optimize outcomes. By standardizing those processes and eliminating variation, they seek to introduce predictability and safety.

With the introduction of consumerism into the healthcare market, there is a growing emphasis on meeting patient expectations, as reflected in patient satisfaction scores. Payers, regulators, and patients are seeking balanced accountability from the provider community. They are demanding efficiency, effectiveness, appropriateness, and personalized and attentive care, each of which is to be measured and publicly reported to achieve transparency. The Joint Commission, through its accreditation process, is often the vehicle through which these expectations are imposed on the healthcare organization.

THE PROVIDER RESPONSE TO IMPROVEMENT INITIATIVES

What has been the provider community's response to these changing and growing expectations? In general, they are seen as illegitimate, arbitrary, and intrusive. The providers see the data on which these initiatives rest as being flawed, naïve, and unfair. For more than a decade, payers, patients, and regulators have been asking the provider community to provide them with data that shows they are receiving safe, reliable, efficient, appropriate, personalized, and affordable care. The provider community has responded by saying that healthcare delivery is too complicated and that they should be trusted to provide necessary and appropriate care free from the oversight of those outside the industry who lack an appreciation of the complexities that accompany clinical decision making.

The judicial system, the legislative process, health maintenance organizations (HMOs), malpractice attorneys, and regulators have entered the void and usurped what had historically been prerogatives of the medical profession. The failure of the physician community to meet the growing expectations for transparency and accountability has eroded a critical element that constitutes professional status, that is an obligation that the profession police itself and hold itself accountable to standards of performance above legal minimums

(O'Conner and Lanning 1992). In seeking to protect individual physician autonomy, physicians are losing group autonomy.

The physician community's response to the report *To Err Is Human* (IOM 1999) was to deny the validity of the conclusion. However, according to Dr. John Kelly (2002), chief patient safety officer at Abington Memorial Hospital, a prospective analysis of patient care outcomes, applying the same methodology used to retrospectively estimate the number of potentially avoidable deaths cited in the report, concluded that the original report actually underestimated by approximately one half the number of avoidable deaths.

Why is it so difficult to engage physicians in initiatives that are designed to improve patient safety and clinical outcomes? I suggest it is because physicians define quality as "the way I take care of patients." All physicians must believe that, in caring for patients, everything they do is as perfect as it can be. I cannot imagine it being otherwise. A physician could not knowingly make decisions on behalf of his patients that he thinks are inappropriate. If your personal physician thinks differently, I strongly urge you to find another physician.

Physicians and Data

This brings up the issue of how physicians respond to data that is used to judge their performance. Because of their medical training, physicians see data as something used in pursuit of identifying absolute truth. As mentioned previously, allopathic medicine seeks to be rooted in the scientific method. The quality of data generally used to assess physician performance is, for the most part, significantly flawed and fails to meet a physician's definition of data. Given that physicians must believe that everything they do is as perfect as it can be, when presented with data that suggest their performance is imperfect, what is their natural conclusion? It is, of course, that the data are flawed. The attempts of most healthcare organizations to improve clinical performance have been, and in many instances continue to be, held hostage to physician demands that the data meet criteria for validity, reliability, and correct scientific methodology.

If this objection can be overcome, the physician's next defense is to impugn the data by suggesting that somehow their patient population was unique. Should those attempts also fail, the final response is to shoot the messenger by challenging the legitimacy of a non-physician administrator's attempt to question the appropriateness of the care provided.

Cultural Barriers

To summarize the physician perspective, the current healthcare delivery system is a culture that

- depends on physician orders;
- rests on personal accountability;
- does not think in terms of processes;
- relies on vigilance and memory;
- places primary emphasis on clinical outcome rather than on balanced accountability that would include efficiency, appropriateness, and quality of patient experience;
- frequently lacks an understanding of medical economics;
- approaches patient care linearly rather than systemically; and
- brings a different set of ethics to clinical decision making.

The Problem of the Apostrophe

Dr. David Eddy (1998) has characterized the point about differing ethics as a problem of the apostrophe, as discussed in Chapter 1. In short, physicians are the patient's advocate, while the healthcare organization is the patients' advocate. An equally valid but separate set of ethics accompanies each of these positions. No one can simultaneously operate in both positions. This creates a natural tension between the healthcare organization and the physicians the organization depends on for success.

I believe these generalizations are valid for traditionalist and boomer physicians. However, these attitudes are being modified by Generation X physicians, who are more willing than their older counterparts to work interdependently and to delegate responsibility. They are more comfortable with the electronic medical record and the use of computerization in support of clinical decision making. The progressive specialization of medical training, together with the growing complexity that accompanies healthcare delivery, makes this a better-adapted approach.

Three Levels of Resistance

Why is it that physicians seem to resist initiatives that are directed at improving patient safety and clinical quality? Resistance to change occurs at three levels (Maurer 1996).

The first level of resistance is factual. The individual seeks logical justification for altering the current way of behaving. Fundamentally, they are requesting the data that say they should alter their behavior. If the strength of the evidence is compelling, they willingly accept the change.

A higher degree of resistance occurs at an emotional level. The individual targeted for change understands the logic, but does not like the implications. Much of the physician resistance to the application of evidence-based guidelines occurs at an emotional level. If preprinted order sets can predictably enhance patient outcomes, what are the implications for the physician? Many physicians perceive that standardizing an approach to patient care diminishes their preeminent position. Since anyone could apply a preprinted order set, the physician might be seen as less necessary. You can overcome emotional resistance only by addressing the emotion, not by continuing to present more fact-based data in hopes of convincing the resister of the correctness of your position. The request for change must be framed in such a way as to allow the physician to perceive that the new behavior will actually enhance her status by freeing her from the mundane task of entering orders, thereby providing time to perform functions for which she is uniquely qualified.

The highest level of resistance is one that occurs at the level of prejudice. This is the hardest type of resistance to overcome, and it fundamentally reflects an absence of trust.

In summary, resistance to change occurs at three levels, where the following questions are asked.

- Level 1: Do I get it?
- Level 2: Do I like it?
- Level 3: Do I like you?

Misidentifying Polarities as Problems

Another point of inertia that accompanies physician resistance to attempts to improve clinical outcomes is the propensity for physicians to misidentify polarities as problems (Johnson 1996). Physicians are inherently "fixers." They identify problems and seek to ameliorate them. Problems represent issues that theoretically have solutions. Decisions are seen as matters of "either/or." Polarities, on the other hand, represent oscillations, wherein either alternative forces you back to reconsider the other. They fundamentally represent "both/and" issues.

There is a tension that exists between the standardization of care processes on the one hand and the perceived need to individualize care on the other. Because there will always be circumstances that make the arbitrary application of standardized approaches to patient care management inappropriate, and because physicians will tend to see this issue as a problem rather than a polarity, they will tend to reject an approach that favors standardization because it is imperfect. If they could perceive this issue as a polarity, they would be able to appreciate that a standardized approach creates predictably better outcomes most of the time and that the challenge is to identify the exceptions that justify deviation from the evidence-based approach.

The data seem clear. Standardized approaches that incorporate evidence-based medicine generally create predictably better outcomes than the individualized artisan approach preferred by physicians. However, because exceptions exist that make the application of standardized approaches sometimes inappropriate to the problem-solving physician, physicians reject this approach in deference to "the perfect care" that they individually apply.

Science vs. the Art of Medicine

The polarity that oscillates between standardization and individualization is a source of great tension within the healthcare community. Currently, the payers, regulators, and legal system are asserting a dominant influence. They insist on standardizing care and seek to penalize those who deviate from the prescribed approach. I am concerned that the *science* of medicine is eclipsing the *art* of medicine. *Curing* is displacing *healing* as the primary consideration. There are four situations in which the rigid adherence to guideline-based medicine may be quite inappropriate (Bujak and Lister 2006):

1. If there are inherently conflicting goals, such as in the areas of pain management, end-of-life care, and the judgment that attends the distinction between "can do" and "should do."
2. If enforcing the application of current knowledge could foreclose on the discovery of new knowledge. Already, the appropriateness of certain measures that are advocated as evidenced-based and appropriate is being called into question by new studies. Excellence is a manifestation of deviant behavior. For something to be truly excellent, it has to exist outside of two standard deviations of the mean or average. For those caregivers who deviate from the prescribed approach and who may discover better ways to manage the patient, the reward

may be exclusion from provider panels and denial of reimbursement. In effect, demands to rigidly adhere to pre-scribed approaches can foreclose on innovation and creativity.

3. If individualizing care. When standardizing care, you risk simultaneously depersonalizing it. In some ways, the patient can become incidental to the practice of medicine. History taking has become automated, and physical examination has been devalued in today's medical training. Today's physicians have become masters at test ordering, where disease and not the patient have become the primary focus of attention. Tests are ordered, diagnostic algorithms are applied, prescribed interventions are recommended, and, too often, individualized appropriateness is not considered. Furthermore, the intense focus on efficiency can further serve to depersonalize care. While efficiency may be appropriately applied to mechanical processes, it should never be applied in the area of human interaction (Woods 2001).

4. If the doctor's presence may modify the healthcare equation. This explains in part the placebo effect, and distinguishes heal-ing from curing, the difference between the art and science of medicine, and the subtleties that separate wisdom from knowl-edge. The physician as healer is threatened by the mechanical scientific and algorithmic approach. The substitution of tech-nology for caretaking can threaten the very soul of medicine.

To quote Dr. Rachel Remen (1996), "too often we even practice medicine this way. Side-by-side, patient and physician focused on the disease, the symptoms, the treatments, never seeing or know-ing each other. The problem gets in the way and we are each alone." The argument here is for the steady advance and application of sci-ence (but not its deification) in a context that equally values and respects individualized human needs.

The push toward emphasis on evidence-based medicine, public reporting of performance data, and pay-for-performance hopefully will not serve to extinguish the art of medicine, devalue transformational doctor-patient relationships, or penalize creativity. Those aspects of the physician's role are intrinsic to the joy and privilege that accompany this unique profession, and they live always in some tension with our best obligation to make rigorous use of "best science."

The current demands for transparency, accountability, and public reporting of data represent a collective challenge to the provider community. How can providers hope to regain or maintain trust and confidence if they cannot demonstrate that they practice state-of-the-art, evidence-based medicine? However, attempts to standardize processes of care significantly and progressively challenge individual physician autonomy. It is at this interface that the majority of resistance in the physician community resides. Unfortunately, the focus on maintaining individual physician autonomy is sacrificing physician group autonomy (Reinertsen 2004).

In the context of balanced accountability, physicians are expected to contribute to the overall quality of patient experience. However, forces within the evolving healthcare industry are moving physicians further away from a personalized doctor-patient relationship. Progressive specialization and economic pressures are pushing physicians to mortgage the doctor-patient relationship in deference to a doctor-disease or a doctor-technology relationship. Generation X physician attitudes amplify this tendency. The progressively more specialized physician manages organs and organ systems. Few physicians actually care for the patient. Hospitalists, who are currently serving to integrate patient care management in the hospital setting, have no presence in the ambulatory sector. When the patient is discharged from the hospital, she returns to the fragmented world of organ system medicine.

SUMMARY

An aging population and the need to manage chronic disease would seem to create a need for more general internists. However, progressively fewer Generation X physicians are selecting general internal medicine as a specialty area. Moreover, the economics of healthcare are bifurcating internal medicine into either an ambulatory-based or a hospital-based specialty. The presence of multisystem disease, the growing complexity of medical care, and the ever-increasing number of medications being prescribed demand that someone serve as the integrator of care. Most healthcare organizations believe in the value of coordinated and integrated patient care. However, the forces of economics and progressive specialization serve to fragment patient care, and the reimbursement system continues to value mechanical interventions of the specialist physician and fails to value the intellectual contribution that accompanies the integration function.

The pursuit of "perfect care" is hindered by a healthcare culture that still emphasizes the primacy of individual physician autonomy with an emphasis on individual accountability, wherein vigilance and memory serve as the basis for delivering safe and quality care. This cultural inertia is reinforced by a tort system that penalizes individuals and hinders the open sharing of information that is useful to the designing of systems and processes of care that hold the promise of enhancing the safety and quality of care.

NOTE

1. Quoted in Mardy Grothe, *Oxymoronica: Paradoxical Wit and Wisdom from History's Greatest Wordsmiths* (New York: HarperCollins, 2004), 30.

REFERENCES

Bujak, J. S., and E. Lister. 2006. "Is the Science of Medicine Trumping the Art of Medicine?" *Physician Executive* 25 (3): 18–21.

Eddy, D. 1998. Presentation on physician leadership to VHA's Physician Leadership Council, Dallas, TX, May 22.

Institute of Medicine (IOM). 1999. *To Err Is Human: Building a Safer Health System*. Washington, DC: National Academies Press.

Johnson, B. 1996. *Polarity Management: Identifying and Managing Unsolvable Problems*. Amherst, MA: HRD Press.

Kelly, J. 2002. Personal communication with the author.

Maurer, R. 1996. *Beyond the Wall of Resistance*. Austin, TX: Bard Books.

O'Conner S. J., and J.A. Lanning. 1992. "The End of Autonomy? Reflections on the Post-Professional Physician." *Healthcare Management Review* 17 (1): 63–72.

Poole, M. S., A. H. Van de Ven, K. Dooley, and M. E. Holmes. 2000. *Organizational Change and Innovation Processes: Theory and Methods for Research*. New York: Oxford University Press.

Reinertsen, J. 2004. "Needless Deaths in Hospitals: Accountability for the Biggest of the Big Dots." Presentation to Meridian Health Board Retreat, Palm Springs, FL, October 22.

Remen, R. 1996. *Kitchen Table Wisdom*. New York: Riverhead Books.

Woods, M. 2001. *Applying Personal Leadership Principles to Healthcare: The DEPO Principle*. Tampa, FL: The American College of Physician Executives.

CHAPTER 6

Engaging Physicians in the Pursuit of Patient Safety and Enhanced Clinical Quality

The chief object of education is not to learn things but to unlearn things.

—G. K. Chesterton[1]

PROVIDE SPRINGBOARD STORIES

When approaching physicians on issues related to changing behavior in support of improvements in patient safety and clinical quality, establishing the proper context is important. In this regard, I believe in the value of springboard stories.

Two of the most powerful stories I have used are the Josie King Story DVD, available from the Josie King Foundation (2007), and an article titled "In Memory of Ben" (Haas 1998). Both of these stories relate to children. In each instance, both the patient and the caregivers were victimized by bad processes that resulted in avoidable and tragic death. Most viewers identify with the powerful emotions portrayed in these stories, and this sets the stage, or provides a springboard, toward establishing the relevance of standardizing care processes.

Springboard stories can move the individual physician beyond a focus preserving his individual autonomy toward a willing commitment to subjugate that autonomy to the appropriate application of defined and reproducible processes. In doing so, he reduces his potential vulnerability and commits to supporting a valued collective objective.

FOCUS ON SAFETY

Attempts to influence physician behavior in support of patient safety and clinical quality should first and foremost focus on the issues related to patient safety. No one can reasonably stand up in a public forum and argue that initiatives designed to enhance patient safety are a bad idea. Moreover, a focus on safety allows the initiator to occupy the moral high ground. You can further argue that you cannot have quality in absence of safety.

On the other hand, seeking to change individual physician behavior through guidelines, preprinted order sets, or other methodologies for standardizing individual patient care is usually accompanied by attempts to defend individual autonomy. Because some exceptions to the universal application of standardized approaches always exist, attempts to reduce variation are invariably victimized by inertia in service of the status quo.

OVERCOME CULTURAL BARRIERS

Dr. Jim Bagian (2003) has identified many cultural elements that resist attempts at enhancing patient safety, including

1. a culture of personal accountability, where the healthcare industry views errors as failings that deserve blame;
2. a blame-and-train mentality, where personal education is the only tool in the improvement toolbox;
3. blind adherence to rules;
4. corrective actions that focus on the individual; and
5. a "no harm, no foul" philosophy.

One way to overcome these barriers is to seek to make "good" better. Too often, attempts at improvement are held hostage to the pursuit of perfection. Exceptions to the rule cannot be used to defend the status quo. Also, focusing first on changing only the few key elements in the patient care process that disproportionately affect the quality of the outcome is preferable. This represents a clinical focus on the Pareto principle, or the 80:20 rule that identifies factors that have a greater impact. Attempts to change too many elements simultaneously complicate the initiative.

Two more cultural elements that present hurdles to the safety agenda are a general lack of awareness and a personal sense of shame that accompanies errors. According to Bagian (2003), a survey at VHA and data from private healthcare organizations show that only 27 percent of respondents agreed that errors were a serious problem, and that 49 percent of respondents felt ashamed by error.

In almost all healthcare organizations, adverse events are categorized on a scale of one to five. A level one incident is one in which no adverse effect is identified, while a level five incident results in death. Most organizations do not even address a potential adverse event unless it is at least a level three. Frequency and severity are inversely related. Close calls are the most frequently encountered experiences. Reporting and studying close calls present a rich opportunity for analyzing current clinical processes of care and correcting them to avoid potentially more serious consequences. You can appreciate that a "no harm, no foul" approach virtually precludes a proactive approach to evaluating close calls. Moreover, reporting near misses transforms a situation from one in which the individual caregiver potentially feels shame into one in which she can be recognized as a heroine.

DISTINGUISH ERRORS, MISHAPS, AND VIOLATIONS FROM SABOTAGE

The healthcare organization needs to distinguish errors, mishaps, and violations from sabotage. An error occurs when someone makes a mistake in carrying out an identified process. For example, one might make a mathematical error in calculating weight-based dosing of a particular medication. A mishap results when someone intending to act in accordance with defined processes becomes distracted or interrupted and thereby forgets to do what was intended or does it improperly or incorrectly.

Violations are a conscious intention to ignore or bypass intended procedure. Physicians frequently make such judgments when they consciously decide to override established procedure because they believe that elements in the current situation justify it. Paradoxically, adverse events occur more frequently in urgent, high-stress situations, when adherence to pre-established procedure would seem to be of greatest benefit. In situations of errors, mishaps, and violations, the individual or individuals involved are fully knowledgeable of the existing procedures and policies that apply. To prescribe further education and training in these circumstances is demeaning and counterproductive. What is required is the identification of the circumstances that would predispose an informed individual to deviate from prescribed processes of care. Eliminating those more primary root causes is key. Except in situations of intentional sabotage, failure to follow established policy is never the primary explanation for adverse events.

Sabotage is a conscious attempt to deviate from prescribed procedure as a way of disrupting or defeating its intention. Assuming that the existing approach is appropriate, sabotage cannot be tolerated.

DEAL WITH DISRUPTIVE PHYSICIANS

It is appropriate at this juncture to discuss the special circumstances that relate to disruptive physician behavior. The Joint Commission has identified failed communication as the most frequent factor contributing to sentinel events (Ramunno 2007). The quality of communication between caregivers is one of the most significant determinants of both patient safety and clinical quality. The disruptive physician is of particular concern because he represents a danger to his patients. The individual often demonstrates disrespectful and demeaning behaviors toward other caregivers, who are intimidated by his aggression. Because they are intimidated, they are less likely to express concerns related to their patients and, in some instances, demonstrate passive-aggressive responses in hopes that the disruptive physician will suffer adverse consequences.

Disruptive physician behavior not only compromises quality of care but also violates organizational core values, reduces joy in the caregiver community, restricts potential, and has significant adverse affect on recruitment and retention (Pfifferling 1999). When healthcare organizations tolerate this behavior, they send a cynical message to their employees. The application of this double standard erodes morale, compromises teamwork, and polarizes various segments that need to work together in pursuit of optimizing patient care.

While nurses, who are employed by the hospital, are required to go through organizational channels to find a remedy, dissatisfied physicians tend to go straight to administration. When administration accommodates or excuses the physician's behavior, it enables the behavior to continue. Certainly, this is an unlevel playing field. Physicians have a higher status than nurses. The expert culture, with its emphasis on power and individual autonomy, is much more aggressive than the more passive affiliative culture that permeates nursing. As employees, nurses are held to behavioral standards that are enforced through the human resources department. Behaving outside the expected norm has consequences. Physicians are still, by and large, not employees of the healthcare organization, and so they stand outside of any organizational structure that is designed to communicate behavioral expectations and to hold employees accountable for deviations from those norms.

While only a small minority of physicians behave badly, a culture of tolerance within the physician community at large contributes to its expression, and the entire organization shares in its consequences.

Disruptive physicians usually follow a consistent pattern. Generally, their disruptive behavior has been long standing. They tend to be very busy and technically competent, but they exhibit a pattern of habitual disregard, especially for those with less status or power. Their behavior tends to be excused in deference to their productivity and clinical competency. If they were disruptive *and* incompetent, they would have been dismissed at the outset.

Disruptive behavior has a number of potential causes, including

- a bullying style that was modeled by early teachers;
- a desire for perfection;
- cultural differences that are becoming more frequent as foreign-trained physicians begin to compensate for the shortfall in physician workforce; and
- individual manifestations of psychiatric disease, personality disorder, or addiction.

Consequences of this behavior include potential organizational liability—because of a threatening work environment or charges of sexual harassment—organizational cynicism, and compromised quality of care. In addition, disruptive behavior undermines practice morale, increases turnover, steals from other productive activities, increases risks for substandard practice, and distresses colleagues.

The ultimate responsibility for dealing with the disruptive physician rests with the governing board. Enforcement is by way of the credentialing process. Responsibility for enforcing behavioral standards should never be left to hospital administration. This presents a no-win situation to the hospital chief executive officer. Appropriate evaluation and enforcement ideally is delegated to the credentialing committee of the medical staff. When that committee is given the choice of either acting appropriately or leaving the responsibility with the board of governors, in my experience, the medical staff will step up to the task. They would rather remain in charge of this activity than defer responsibility to an outside group.

Every healthcare organization and its related medical staff need to develop an explicit policy that relates to physician behavior. This policy needs to merge interpersonal behavioral expectations with clinical practice expectations. It must set standards of conduct, especially when it may affect quality of care. When dealing with the disruptive physician, follow a specific procedure:

- Episodes must be fully documented.
- The circumstances should be fully assessed.
- Those directly involved or witnessing the episode should provide their perspective.
- The physician must be confronted and allowed to tell her side of the story.

While extenuating circumstances might make the behavior understandable, disrespectful and disruptive expressions can never be tolerated. That is, the behavior might be understood, but its inappropriateness is nonnegotiable. Expectations for future behavior and consequences for violation of those expectations must be explicitly stated. Resources should be identified that might support the physician in his attempts to control his behavior. The approach can be summarized as evaluating what you can do *for* the physician rather than *to* the physician. The individual in question might be having personal difficulties outside of the professional work environment. Support with family stresses, financial difficulties, and, at times, addiction hold the potential of rehabilitating and salvaging a potentially productive career.

REDESIGN PATIENT CARE PROCESSES AND SYSTEMS

Bagian (2003) has outlined critical elements that support an effective patient safety system. Framing the initiative as a learning opportunity and not as an accountability system is important. A non-punitive, confidential reporting system that allows people to remain anonymous is essential, as is reporting close calls. All reports should emphasize narratives. Failure to follow procedure is never an explanation for an adverse patient event. Defining the circumstances that promote deviation from known policy and ameliorating those circumstances are more critical. Interdisciplinary review teams need to be established. Giving prompt feedback to individuals involved reinforces the potential for learning. Remember that the data collection is an attempt to identify vulnerabilities and is not merely an exercise in statistics.

Patient care processes need to be redesigned in a way to reduce primary reliance on memory and vigilance. Those involved in engineering safe practices identify memory and vigilance as the two weakest links in the safe practice chain. Processes should be designed to simplify and standardize. Checklists and forcing functions are important elements. At an organizational level, it is important to increase feedback, emphasize teamwork, drive out fear, demonstrate leadership's commitment, and improve direct communication.

There is an interesting contrast between safety initiatives in industries that focus intensely on safety—such as commercial aviation and the nuclear power industry—and healthcare. Commerical aviation and industries like it rely on redundant systems to achieve maximum safety (Weick and Sutcliffe 2001). The value of redundancy stands in contrast to an emphasis on efficiency that dominates work redesign efforts within the healthcare industry, which is challenged by progressively shrinking profit margins.

The challenge is to figure out how safety initiatives can achieve a status equivalent to that of operating room sterile technique. No one challenges the appropriateness of and insistence upon sterile technique in the operating room setting. How can similar standards be applied to all other areas of patient care? Put another way, as scientists, why can physicians not apply science to the journey toward achieving perfect care? They need to demonstrate the will. Issues of patient safety must be made nonnegotiable.

The growing presence of intensivists and hospitalists will significantly contribute to enhancements in patient safety and clinical quality. These hospital-based physicians have an intrinsic appreciation for an interdisciplinary approach to patient care that incorporates predictable and standardized processes. In addition, these physicians can be contractually rewarded for incorporating a best practice approach. Having patients cared for by fewer physicians who are specifically trained in acute care medicine represents a meaningful improvement over the "any willing provider" approach that has been the historical norm.

The Institute for Healthcare Improvement's emphasis on bundling interventions has been a significant advance in the journey toward enhanced patient safety (Schraag 2008). The ventilator bundle can all but eliminate ventilator-associated pneumonia. The surgical infection prevention bundle significantly reduces the frequency of surgery-related infections. The sepsis bundle holds the promise of improving the outcome in this group of critically ill patients. The emphasis on hand washing and the application of a central-line bundle markedly reduce the frequency of nosocomial infections and central-line sepsis, respectively.

MANAGE MEDICATION PROCEDURES

Managing medications is essential to any program that addresses patient safety. Given the high number of medications prescribed to hospitalized patients, it is easy to see why medication errors represent the greatest potential source of avoidable harm. A number of initiatives are being applied in this important area. The decentralization of pharmacy with an emphasis on placing clinically trained pharmacists in the patient care areas holds immense promise. Having clinical pharmacists available to physicians, nurses, and patients brings their expertise to bear. They can review the appropriateness of prescriptions, and help guide the physician, teach the nurse, and educate the patient regarding medications. Clinical pharmacists can be the most appropriate individuals for performing medication reconciliation. Ample data document that the times of greatest patient risk occur when patients are shifted from one level of care to another (Pronovost et al. 2003). At these times, when handoffs are necessary, the greatest number of mistakes is made, hence the value of medication reconciliation in service of patient safety. The insistence on entering patient data such as age, weight, allergy history, and level of kidney function are integral to safe medication management practices. Sophisticated software programs can prompt the pharmacists to recognize the potential for adverse medication events before dispensing newly prescribed medication.

Adverse medication events can originate when prescribing, dispensing, or administering. At the prescribing level, the focus should be on clarity, as it relates to physician handwriting, and the appropriateness of the prescription from a medical perspective. In all but the most emergent of situations, it is imperative to check for the appropriateness of the drug, its dose, and the route of administration before the first dose is given. Regarding administration, the nurse must confirm that she is giving the right drug, the right dose, by the right route, at the right time to the right patient. Bar-coding medications can significantly affect medication safety at this level.

Another valuable way to reduce medication errors is medication reconciliation. The importance of this function has been emphasized by the Joint Commission, which has established it as a functional requirement for accreditation. Unfortunately, medication reconciliation is rarely performed as intended. Narrowly trained physician subspecialists feel ill-prepared to reconcile the multiple medications that most patients receive. The most appropriate physician to perform this function would be the patient's primary care physician, but these physicians are progressively disappearing from the hospital setting. While pharmacists would appear well qualified to perform this function, they might not know whether a particular medication was prescribed for an "off-label" purpose.

By default, in most organizations, medicine reconciliation has been assigned to nurses. This is inappropriate, in my opinion. Nurses are not by training or experience prepared to serve this function. Reconciling medications that are being taken in the ambulatory setting can often take several hours, and doing so further removes the nurse from face-to-face patient contact. Too often, medication reconciliation is a perfunctory exercise that appears to comply with regulations but falls far short of its intended contribution.

Fortunately, there is good news regarding medication errors. The expanding presence of hospitalists and the decentralization of clinical pharmacists, together with the application of appropriate software programs, will significantly reduce adverse prescribing. Several other practices are also improving this situation, including attention to packaging and storing, standardization of concentration, a primary focus on medications administered intravenously, and an emphasis on those medicines most frequently involved in serious adverse events (e.g., pain medications, anticoagulants, insulin, and antibiotics).

CREATE RAPID RESPONSE TEAMS

Creating rapid response teams also enhances patient safety. Rapid response teams identify patients at risk prior to coding. In many ways, the need to create rapid response teams is a response to the progressive disappearance of physicians from the hospital. Surgeons prefer to spend time in the operating room, leaving pre- and post-operative care to physician assistants, while general internists and family practitioners prefer to remain in the ambulatory setting. A task orientation compromises the nurse's ability to closely assess the patient. Over time, an increasing number of hospital-based physicians could make rapid response teams less necessary.

UNDERSTAND PHYSICIAN DYNAMICS

With regard to engaging physicians in safety and quality initiatives, refer back to some of the dynamics discussed in previous chapters. Recall how skeptics and mismatchers can quickly identify potentially inappropriate applications of standardized processes. Because the proposed solution is not perfect, physicians often reject it, despite the probability of creating improved aggregated outcomes. "Perfect" becomes the enemy of "better." Remember that resistance often occurs at an emotional level and that status-conscious physicians needing to preserve their sense of authority and control will resist standardization because they perceive an erosion of their authority and a diminished sense of importance. Finally, all new behaviors are clumsy and require more time and effort to apply. It must be clear that the deliverable justifies the effort.

So how might you proceed? First, encourage open and clear communication, both verbal and written. Pre-brief and debrief. Accomplish this with a preprocedure "timeout" or huddle and a postprocedure summary of findings and implications. Invest the time in performing failure mode effect analyses (FMEAs). These exercises, together with an emphasis on evaluating close calls, can help you anticipate areas that require redesign. Incorporate cognitive aids and checklists as ways of preventing errors of omission. Eliminate the "who is at fault" question as the initial response to an adverse event. Finally, a commitment to safety and quality must be led by the board, healthcare organization administration, and physician champions.

SUMMARY

According to Jim Bagian (2003), initiatives that address safety and quality are not about tabulating errors. Rather, they are about identifying vulnerabilities. Analysis, action, and feedback are the keys. Patient safety and quality are about prevention and not punishment. Cultural change is the key, and that will take time. Safety is indeed the foundation upon which quality is built. Structural changes, like employing intensivists and hospitalists, will go a long way toward building safe, quality medical practice. In addition, as more physicians are employed, we will find physicians serving in management roles at the head of service lines, where they will be supplied with data that can support the kinds of structure and process changes that will drive the safety and quality initiatives toward "perfect care." Fundamentally, creating a safe patient care environment is a matter of *will* more than *resources*. We get what we accept, and what we accept sets the standard. What would the response be if the chief financial officer only billed patients 90 percent of the time? By analogy, how can we accept applying appropriate patient care less frequently than it should be?

NOTE

1. Quoted in Mardy Grothe, *Oxymoronica: Paradoxical Wit and Wisdom from History's Greatest Wordsmiths* (New York: HarperCollins, 2004), 171.

REFERENCES

Bagian, J. 2003. *Safety—A Systems Approach*. Presentation in Baltimore, MD, November 7.

Haas, D. 1998. "In Memory of Ben." *Risk Management Reports* 25 (12). [Online article; retrieved 2/1/08.] www.riskreports.com/protected/archive/rmr1298.html

Josie King Foundation. 2007. "Foundation Programs." [Online information; retrieved 2/1/08.] www.josieking.org

Pfifferling, J. H. 1999. "The Disruptive Physician: A Quality of Professional Life Factor." *Physician Executive* 25 (2): 56–61.

Pronovost, P., B. Weast, M. Schwarz, R. M. Wyskiel, S. N. Milanovich, S. Berenholtz, T. Dorman, and P. Lipsett. 2003. "Medication Reconciliation: A Practical Tool to Reduce the Risk of Medication Errors." *Journal of Critical Care* 18 (4): 201–5.

Ramunno, L. D. 2007. "Hospital Governing Boards and Quality: A Call to Responsibility." Presentation at Main Health/QHR Governance Conference, Bar Harbor, ME, October 13.

Schraag, J. 2008. "Bundling Is Better, Experts Say." *Infection Control Today*, January 24.

Weick, K. D., and J. K. Sutcliffe. 2001. *Managing the Unexpected: Assuring High Performance in an Age of Complexity*. San Francisco: Jossey Bass.

CHAPTER 7

Why Physicians and Healthcare Organizations Distrust Each Other

Unhappiness is not knowing what we want and killing ourselves to get it.

—Don Herold[1]

Everyone seems to acknowledge that physicians and healthcare administrators distrust each other. Why is this distrust a universal occurrence? This chapter seeks to provide the answer.

A DIFFERENCE IN PERCEPTION

Perception is reality. A person's behavior makes perfect sense from his point of view. When I am teaching a seminar, I often present a slide that simultaneously depicts both an old woman and a young woman. I give the audience only a few seconds to look at the slide. If they have never seen this slide before, in the brief time allotted they are unlikely to identify both of the figures. After turning off the slide, I ask the audience to make a series of choices on behalf of the individual they have seen, based on her age. The choices are polarizingly distinct. For example, I ask them to choose a television program for this individual to watch: a recent music video or reruns of "The Lawrence Welk Show." I ask them to plan a vacation for this person: going scuba diving in Cozumel or taking a cruise with the Glenn Miller Orchestra. By a show of hands, the audience indicates their specific choices.

The audience will look around the room and see that a significant number of individuals did not agree with their choices. Perhaps a majority wonders, Why do they disagree? What do they see that I missed? Perhaps others quickly conclude that those who are in disagreement are wrong, because the answers are so obvious. I believe that the picture of the old woman and a young woman represents a metaphor for misunderstanding that can occur in any relationship. In a healthcare setting, rather than ask why someone disagrees with our conclusions (which seem so clear based on our own perception), we tend to conclude that the other person is either incompetent or self-serving. In any event, those who disagree with us are not to be trusted. We are predisposed to argue over who is right and who is wrong rather than embarking on a course of enhanced mutual understanding. It is through a willingness to simultaneously practice advocacy and inquiry that we are open to an enhanced understanding, a broader appreciation of the complexity of the issue, and an opportunity to synthesize new and creative possibilities.

Overcoming Differences in Opinion

To enhance mutual understanding, you essentially advocate for your position. Explain what you think and why you think it. Then, build a bridge toward greater understanding by acknowledging that the other person's conclusions must make equally good sense to her. Ask her to explain what she thinks and why she thinks it. It is through this dialogue that you create the capacity for enhanced mutual understanding. In addition, you come to better appreciate and understand your own position. Have you ever tried to explain something, and while you are explaining it, you actually come to understand it differently than you did at the outset? The act of trying to explain something causes us to see with greater understanding and clarity. This approach significantly reduces any propensity to distrust through misunderstanding, assumption, or biased misinterpretation.

A DIFFERENCE IN ASSUMPTIONS

Another exercise that I like to conduct is presenting to the audience a list of 10 words, all of which have something to do with sleep. I give them only 10 seconds to look at this list, and then I ask them to write down as many of the words as they can remember. Invariably, a majority will write down the word "sleep" even though it was not on the list. There is an assumption that sleep was on the list. This exercise demonstrates how frequently we fail to adequately communicate. The listener assumes he has understood what the speaker has said, while the speaker presumes that what she has said has been understood as intended. Assuming underlies a significant amount of misunderstanding. This failure to communicate with absolute clarity often leads to unanticipated results. When this occurs, the participants again mistakenly conclude that the other party is not trustworthy.

I then ask the participants to engage in a third exercise. I quickly ask them to take a large sheet of paper, fold it in half, and tear off the right upper corner. Intentionally hurrying through the exercise, I then instruct them to again fold the paper in half, but this time to tear off the right lower corner. Once again, I request them to fold the paper in half, but this time to tear off the left upper corner. I then tell the audience to unfold their paper and hold it high above their heads while they look around the room. It is amazing to see the wide variety of snowflakes that are produced from these sequence commands.

Because so few of the snowflakes match, I ask the audience whose fault it is that they could not successfully follow this list of commands. Many respond that it is my fault for not giving clear enough instructions. I quickly acknowledge that if creating a specific snowflake was my intention, I should have given very explicit instructions and even provided a sample of my vision for how the final product should look. However, I point out that no one stopped me to ask me for directions that were more specific. Many of them were unsure how to fold the paper and which corner to tear. However, they saw that others in the room were busy folding and tearing, and so they assumed that the others must understand the instructions. They did not want to give the impression that they were not paying attention or were too slow to understand, so they did not ask for clearer directions.

OVERCOMING MISUNDERSTANDING

These three exercises—the old woman/young woman illusion, the word game, and the snowflake exercise—demonstrate some of the more frequent experiences that cause people to conclude that others are either incompetent or untrustworthy. They certainly occur with great frequency in conversations between physicians and hospital administrators.

Overcoming misunderstanding is a prerequisite for generating new possibilities. Facilitated dialogue, in which each party advocates for his position while seeking to understand the other's position, allows for self-discovery that can alter existing beliefs and change behaviors.

Personality Preferences

It is also important to appreciate how individuals pursue sense-making. Individuals have preferences, based on their personalities, that predispose them to selectively perceive and appreciate things that are important to them. Ned Herrmann (1996) distinguishes four distinctive personality preference styles. Some individuals are predisposed to analyze, while others organize, socialize, or strategize as preferred approaches to making sense of their environment. No person is all of one or the other, but certain tendencies predominate.

Physicians' choice of specialty practice is often a reflection of their personality preferences. General surgeons, radiologists, and emergency room physicians emphasize the analytical. These individuals like to quantify things and focus on the information necessary to make logical and rational decisions. Neurologists, pathologists, nephrologists, and gastroenterologists often have a predisposition to organize. Organizers establish procedures, get things done, make plans, and are reliable, neat, and timely.

Relationships are very important to socializers, who are sensitive to others, like to teach, and are supportive, expressive, and emotional. Feelings are very important to socializers. Pediatricians, family practice physicians, obstetricians, and psychiatrists reflect this preference.

Infectious disease physicians, oncologists, and some pathologists are often big-picture thinkers. Their work requires an ability to think broadly in terms of differential diagnosis and multisystem disease. These strategizers are characterized as individuals who infer, imagine, speculate, take risks, break rules, like surprises, and are impetuous and curious.

To effectively communicate, it is critical to speak in the language of the receiver—to be in tune to the parts of your message that are important to the receiver, based on her personality preference. Emphasizing relationships and emotions to someone who is predominantly analytical is not likely to capture his attention. Similarly, failing to address the relationship and emotional consequences of logical decisions creates push back from those who emphasize social interaction. In a similar fashion, big-picture thinkers feel tethered by those organizers who are risk averse, respectful of policy, and detail focused. The organizers, in turn, accuse the big-picture thinkers of having their heads in the clouds.

Successful communicators appreciate the other's individual stylistic preference. It is imperative to package your information in a way that addresses the implications of your message that are most meaningful to the receiver. Failure to do so would be the equivalent of speaking in a foreign language that the other person does not understand.

When the person being addressed does not understand the language, it is common for the speaker to repeat the words louder and slower. However, it is far more effective to translate the message into a language that the receiver understands. The conversation that is most effective when engaging a neurosurgeon is a very different conversation from one involving a pediatrician. How you package your message, the points you emphasize, your rationale, and the impact of your message must be distinctive if you are to successfully influence the listener.

Perception is an act of creation. We are able to perceive only what we are programmed to receive. We recognize only those things for which we have pre-existing mental maps. Learning is a shifting of where it is we choose to pay attention. In the book *Crucial Conversations*, Patterson and colleagues (2002) describe how individuals respond to others. The basic sequence is as follows. We take in information through our senses and simultaneously "apply our story"—that is, we instantly interpret or judge the information. How we interpret or judge that information triggers an emotion appropriate to that judgment. Based on that emotion, we then act on the information.

Our existing triggers and filters influence this process (Atchison and Bujak 2001). We are predisposed to recognize those elements in our environment that reaffirm our existing beliefs and assumptions about how things are. We are equally predisposed to ignore data elements that would contradict our current way of making sense. The information is not objective information, but rather information colored by our pre-existing prejudices, biases, and beliefs. Our emotions are triggered by our interpretation as a reflection of our personal needs and expectations, not by the source of the external data per se.

CHANGING EXPECTATIONS

The expectations we carry with us are, for the most part, inherited from our cultures. Our parents, relatives, teachers, ministers, friends, colleagues, and other influencers create expectations that we tend to accept at face value. Because physicians and hospital administrators carry a separate set of operating assumptions, beliefs, and attitudes about how the healthcare system should operate, they are each predisposed to see and interpret the data differently and therefore to behave in ways conditioned by their expectations. It is imperative to distinguish between our assumptions, our feelings, and the facts.

When challenged by the need to respond to a changing external environment, ask yourself the following questions (Zander and Zander 2000):

- What assumptions am I making that cause me to see what I see?
- What might I invent, that hasn't yet been invented, that would give me other choices?

Our view of the world is an invention. If we change our assumptions, beliefs, and attitudes, then we change what we see, how we react, and how we behave. What are your limiting beliefs?

Ben and Rosamund Zander suggest that we are raised in a world of measurement. The assumption is that life is about staying alive and surviving in a world of scarcity and peril. It is a world of competition. When our expectations are not met, we react with an array of negative emotions.

Anthony DeMello (1990) suggests that the observer self, or "I," needs to be aware of the subjective self, or "me." He suggests that all emotions arise from within the subjective self in response to how our needs are either being met or not being met. Throughout our lives, individuals in positions of authority (parents, teachers, clergy, coaches, mentors, etc.) have set our expectations in the form of *shoulds* and *oughts* that we accept as the way our world is supposed to be. Our emotions are a response to whether these expectations are being met. When the "I" as an objective observer can sense that the "me" is experiencing emotion, she can examine the subjective expectation that is or isn't being met, which is the source of the emotion. Others don't cause our emotions; they are consequent to our own invented expectations. DeMello sees values such as acknowledgment, appreciation, and affection as drugs that we've been given since early childhood to which we have become addicted. We have been conditioned to desire those rewards and become disappointed, angry, or devalued when they are not forthcoming. Just becoming aware acts to diffuse the emotion and allows us to experience life as it unfolds in the meaningful present.

I mention this here in hopes of provoking you to appreciate that who we are is an invention; that we are preconditioned to interpret our world according to imposed expectations; and that most of our frustrations, disappointments, and conflicts are really consequent to a failure to achieve the expectations that these fantasies create. These elements underlie the tension that exists in relationships between physicians and hospital administrators.

SUMMARY

Physicians and hospital administrators distrust each other because they interpret information through differing frames of reference. Physicians perceive things linearly, have a short time frame of reference, and act as the patient's advocate. Administrators must apply a systems perspective, plan for the long-term, and serve as the patients' advocate. Each is so convinced that their view is "right" that for the other not to see it similarly must be indication that they are either unable to see or choose not to see. In either case, they are not to be trusted. Reality is created by perceptions, and individuals selectively see what reinforces their preexisting biases while failing to see what challenges those perceptions. Our expectations frame what we see and what we cannot see. Trust is built through revealing ourselves, by ensuring that we communicate explicitly, and by being transparent in stating our position and the rationale that supports it while simultaneously inquiring as to the rationale that guides the position of the other.

NOTE

1. Quoted in Mardy Grothe, *Oxymoronica: Paradoxical Wit and Wisdom from History's Greatest Wordsmiths* (New York: HarperCollins, 2004), 177.

REFERENCES

Atchison, T., and J. Bujak. 2001. *Leading Transformational Change: The Physician-Executive Partnership*. Chicago: Health Administration Press.

DeMello, A. 1990. *Awareness: The Perils and Opportunities*. New York: Image.

Herrmann, N. 1996. *The Whole Brain Business Book*. New York: McGraw-Hill.

Patterson, K., J. Grenny, R. McMillan, and A. Switzler. 2002. *Crucial Conversations: Tools for Talking When Stakes Are High*. New York: McGraw-Hill.

Zander, R. S., and B. Zander. 2000. *The Art of Possibility*. New York: Penguin Books.

CHAPTER 8

The Healthcare Leader as an Agent of Change: Challenges and Consequences

And those who were seen dancing were thought to be insane by those who could not hear the music.

—Friedrich Wilhelm Nietzsche[1]

If you plot the passage of time along the horizontal axis against the pace of change up the vertical axis, the result is an asymptotic curve (Russell 1998). The relationship is hyperbolic and suggests that the pace of change is occurring at an exponential rate. The point at which the curve rounds the bend and heads north is "the point of singularity." At this point, the pace of change is occurring so rapidly that the equation that plots the curve generates results that are so close to infinity that the points become indistinguishable and, hence, singular. The point of singularity related to the pace of change is projected to occur no later than the middle of this century. At this point, it will be virtually impossible to identify change. Everything will be in a constant state of transition.

This relationship appears to hold no matter what the frame of reference is. You could be plotting the pace of change of communication technology or the evolution of the mammalian species. In either event, the relationship is suggestively exponential. In a similar way, the doubling time of knowledge is accelerating.

Currently, the rate is estimated to be somewhere between three and four years.

Medical school is a four-year curriculum. Most residency training programs are at least three years long, and fellowships can range from an additional one to three years. Given the rapid progression of change and the acceleration in knowledge, a long period of training seems frustratingly irrelevant. Advancing technology is poised to progressively challenge current medical practice. Any failure to remain current threatens to render the practitioner obsolete.

IDENTIFY YOUR MISSION AND PURPOSE

This phenomenon requires that all healthcare professionals be able to separate the essence of who they are and what they do from the forms in which they are currently being made manifest. Whatever you are doing today, you will not be doing tomorrow. New technology is constantly challenging the competency and relevance of everyone. If you are what you do, and you do not, then you are not!

The following is a common progression in the life of an evolving gastroenterologist. Having passed general internal medicine boards, the individual chooses to pursue gastroenterology as a specialty. At this point, he no longer desires to treat issues related to general internal medicine, such as diabetes, congestive heart failure, or hypertension. Having successfully passed his gastroenterology boards, he might choose to focus on colonoscopy as an area of special expertise. At this point, even though he is a board-certified gastroenterologist, he may refuse to take care of patients with liver disease or small bowel disease, preferring instead to spend the day doing colonoscopies. What would happen to this individual if a test were developed that, with great specificity and sensitivity, could identify patients with colon cancer? Since the vast majority of colonoscopies are diagnostic and without significant findings, the economic security of his present practice style would become significantly challenged.

In an analogous fashion, what is the future of an interventional cardiologist subsequent to the development of noninvasive imaging of the coronary circulation? The majority of diagnostic heart catheterizations reveal an absence of significant disease. Just as stents have reduced the frequency of coronary artery bypass graft surgery, medications and initiatives focused on prevention hold the promise of reversing and preventing plaque-related coronary artery disease and significantly reducing the need for interventional coronary angiography.

When everything around you is changing at an ever-more rapidly progressing rate, what remains immutable? This question challenges everyone. In this substance-versus-form issue, you must identify the essence of who you are and the purpose of your work. There is a subtle but meaningful distinction between the terms "mission" and "purpose." Your purpose ideally represents your vocational calling, which remains constant. Mission, on the other hand, is the way in which your purpose is currently being made manifest. The mission may change, while the purpose remains constant. As the seasons change, an individual changes his wardrobe, but the wearer of the clothes is unchanged.

POSITION YOUR ORGANIZATION

Given this rapid and accelerating pace of change, those in positions of leadership need to position their organization for sustainability. A story is told that when Wayne Gretzky was asked how he managed to score more goals than any other hockey player, he is said to have replied, "It is because I skate to where the puck is *going to be.*" He did not choose to skate to where the puck *was* and certainly not to where the puck *had been.* In an analogous fashion, organizational leaders must seek to position their organization where they believe "the puck is going to be." Failure to do so places the organization at a significant disadvantage. To accomplish this, leaders must serve in the capacity of change agent. Adaptability becomes the key to sustainability.

In a world that is changing this rapidly, the future is more than unpredictable. It is unknowable. Therefore, leaders need to develop robust strategies. "Robust adaptive strategies willingly sacrifice the focus, apparent certainty, efficiency, and coordination that traditional strategies provide for the sake of flexibility and a higher probability of success" (Beinhocker 1999). Put another way, what is the current value of a five-year plan?

A rapidly changing world belongs to the entrepreneur. In this context, an entrepreneur is defined as an individual willing to act on less-than-perfect information. Entrepreneurs have a great tolerance for risk and are confident in their own intuitive judgment. Contrast that approach with the usual approach within the healthcare industry, wherein certain knowledge is a precondition to action.

When an organizational leader seeks to shift the dominant paradigm, what percentage of individuals within the organization can see excitement and possibility in novelty? The answer lies somewhere in the range of 15 percent (Rogers 1995). When managing for consensus is the preferred avenue for decision making, transformational change is impossible in the absence of an immediate and significant threat. In effect, only heretics create change.

PROMOTE ADAPTABILITY

If this is the case, how does a leader effectively position the organization for adaptability? The complexity scientist Ralph Stacey would suggest that this is done by introducing a controlled amount of anxiety into the organization (Zimmerman 1998). Too little anxiety causes those within the organization to be too comfortable to engage in the change process. Too much anxiety creates a hectic and stressful environment, wherein effective change is more difficult. Stacey would suggest that introducing a controlled amount of anxiety could be accomplished by adjusting four significant variables:

- *Selectively control the amount of new information introduced to the group.* There must be enough information to challenge the status quo, and yet not so much information as to create chaos.

- *Invest in organizational diversity.* Diversity of opinion and diversity of perspective lead to a consideration of an enriched array of possibilities.
- *Connect the diverse elements.* Having diversity is not enough unless the diverse elements are effectively connected. Conversation and dialogue nurture self-organization and the emergence of potential solutions.
- *Effectively distribute power within the organization.* When power is centered primarily at the leadership level, the command-and-control nature of the organization impairs its adaptability. If power is too decentralized throughout the organization, then it becomes difficult to focus specific initiatives.

Tom Atchison (Atchison and Bujak 2001) suggests that the word "change" should be seen as a red flag. His point is that individuals change all of the time. When they find themselves in a position of understanding, wanting, and controlling the change, the change is perceived as an opportunity. People do not mind changing in this setting. People do, however, resist being changed. This happens when individuals find themselves in circumstances they do not understand, want, or control. In a similar way, Atchison would suggest that change is most feasible when individuals within the organization are at a midpoint between the extremes of being happy and being angry. When people are very happy, they are not inclined to change because they are content. When significant anger is the dominant emotion, people are unwilling to change because they cannot get beyond their own anger. This fits nicely into Stacey's (Zimmerman 1998) scheme of how best to promote adaptability.

PRIORITIZE ORGANIZATIONAL VALUES

Given the accelerating pace of change, organizational leaders must prioritize organizational values. By that I mean create a hierarchy of relative importance in relation to the various change initiatives that may be occurring simultaneously. Without clearly defining the hierarchy of organizational values, individuals do not have a clear understanding of which initiatives should take precedence. Invariably, there are times when busy individuals are faced with the need to choose between two behaviors. While both may be clearly important, they cannot be performed simultaneously, and it should be clear which of the two is more important.

For example, nurses are frequently confronted with competing priorities. Imagine that there is one half hour before the end of a nurse's shift. She has yet to complete her charting. A family, with whom the nurse needs to discuss a patient's illness and its implications, appears. Only one half hour is left to shift report, and the nurse's charting is incomplete. Discussing the implications of a patient's illness for both the patient and the patient's family is an essential element of the nurse's role, and this is the first opportunity she has had to engage the family. What should she do? Both are important. How does the organization help to prioritize her decision making?

The current emphasis on creating an electronic medical record significantly challenges today's nurses. New activities that accompany documentation, regulatory requirements, concerns over controlling labor costs that affect staffing ratios, the growing complexity of medical care, and the increasing acuity and shortened length of stay of most inpatients present real challenges. Nurse-patient contact time is progressively lessening, and this significantly affects professional satisfaction. Moreover, nurses are becoming "task doers." The lifestyle realities that promote 12-hour shifts further erode continuity of patient care and may significantly contribute to compromises in patient safety.

Physicians are constantly in a hurry. Doctors and nurses find it progressively more difficult, if not impossible, to make patient care rounds together. What then becomes the vehicle for communicating? What are the critical elements related to managing a specific patient? Care is becoming progressively depersonalized, technical, and fragmented.

Given these dynamics, there is a need to appreciate that in a world where everything is changing at a rapid rate, shared values and shared purpose are unchangeable. Such purpose and values need to be explicitly defined and prioritized to establish the foundation on which trust, collaboration, and meaningful partnerships can be built.

IMPLICATIONS OF BEING A CHANGE AGENT

What are the implications of serving as a change agent? The answer is of biblical proportions. Change agents seek to shift the paradigm in promotion of transformational change. All groups act to defend the status quo. All groups are most responsive to their most powerful constituent group. That group, by definition, is disproportionately served by the existing paradigm. To advocate for change is to challenge that group's preeminent position. For that reason, there is a predictable sequence of responses that challenge individuals who would shift the paradigm.

The initial response is ridicule. The shared belief system among the group is so strong that presuming to challenge one of those beliefs or existing paradigms evokes ridicule. The next level of response is to marginalize the individual. If these fail to silence the individual, the final step would be to excommunicate them from the group.

Since only a small minority of individuals can imagine positive consequences to transformational changes, the majority will actively reject the idea. In effect, then, the fate of all change agents is to be rejected by the very group they seek to advantage. Prophets never enter the promised land. Most change agents, however, are compelled to act on their passions. They cannot *not* do what they feel called to do. Change agents are compelled by the journey and not by the need to reach a specific destination.

Healthcare leaders—those I know who have had an effect on the industry—all tell the same story. At one point in their careers, they became disillusioned with the distractions, competitions, and progressive frustrations that had come to dominate their work life. They were tired of fighting with payers, regulators, other healthcare organizations, physicians, and politicians. They were especially tired of playing it safe and trying to please all constituents. They decided that if they were going to go down, they would go down for something they cared about. For one, it was Planetree; for another, pursuit of the Malcolm Baldrige Award; for a third, it was Six Sigma and Toyota's Lean Production methodology; and for another, it was the creation of a community cancer center. At the point of their commitment, a paradox occurred. In choosing to pursue their passion and to let go of the potential consequences, they found a majority within the organization willing to support it energetically. In my view, people who work in healthcare are eager for leadership to articulate that their work is about more than the money.

JOURNEYING TOWARD THE FUTURE

To appreciate how this all fits together, it is important to understand the nature of the creative process (Fritz 1999). The essence of the creative process is the capacity to simultaneously visualize an idealized future and have an honest assessment of current reality. The tension that exists between *what is* and *what might be* drives the process closer to the vision. This dynamic highlights the importance of vision to effective leadership and simultaneously challenges leadership to see current circumstances as they really are supported by meaningful metrics.

The journey toward the future requires that the *what* of the proposal be explicitly defined. The *why*, or the compelling rationale, must be passionately communicated. The *who*, those who would participate, must be matched to the values hierarchy that will define the character of the enterprise. This values hierarchy is how all decisions will be made going forward. The *when* establishes a timeline, and the *where* establishes the boundaries that will contain the initiative. Finally, specific *metrics* must be identified through which progress will be gauged and success measured. This foundation must be established with explicit clarity before moving toward the *how* that will guide the journey toward the vision. In my experience, healthcare organization and physician partnerships rarely explicitly define the enterprise as outlined above, leaving the what to be defined by individual assumption, the metrics uncertain, the values unspecified, and the how being jumped to immediately.

SUMMARY

In summary, living in a world that is changing at an ever-more accelerating pace demands that leaders serve in the capacity of change agent. It is imperative to anticipate the future and to invest in the organization's human capital and their ability to adapt. What binds the workforce together is shared purpose and values. These can remain immutable as technology and other forces act to transform the ways the shared purpose and values become expressed. Leading to manifest a transcendent purpose is the way that agents of change can overcome the inertia that accompanies all organizations when confronted with the challenges of adapting to change. Because all change is clumsy, an energizing and inspiring vision must be communicated and modeled so that all can continue to experience meaning and purpose in their work.

NOTE

1. WritersMugs Gallery, accessed online June 1, 2008, www.writersmugs.com/quotes.php?day=169.

REFERENCES

Atchison, T., and J. Bujak. 2001. *Leading Transformational Change: The Physician-Executive Partnership*. Chicago: Health Administration Press.

Beinhocker, E. D. 1999. "Robust Adaptive Strategies." *Sloan Management Review* 40 (3): 95–106.

Fritz, R. 1999. *The Path of Least Resistance for Managers: Designing Organizations to Succeed.* San Francisco: Berrett-Koehler.

Rogers, E. M. 1995. *Diffusions of Innovations.* New York: Free Press.

Russell, P. 1998. *Waking Up in Time: Finding Inner Peace in Times of Accelerating Change.* Novato: Origin Press.

Zimmerman, B. 1998. *Edgeware.* Irving, TX: VHA, Inc.

CHAPTER 9

Reflections

The love we give away is the only love we keep.
—Elbert Hubbard[1]

My personal passion is to contribute in any way that I can to increasing a sense of joy in the healthcare professions. Currently, physician professional satisfaction is at an all-time low (Terrell 2007). Physicians too often advise their children not to pursue a career in medicine and frequently regret their own choice to have done so. When I ask a physician audience why it is that professional satisfaction is so low, a number of explanations are offered in response. The list usually identifies causal factors outside of the individual physician. However, when I ask the physicians, "Who is responsible for your happiness?" the reply is invariably, "I am." This is a pivotal dynamic that reflects where the individual assigns the locus of control. As long as the locus of control is placed outside of the individual, that person is a victim. He can never be happy until external agencies "get their act together" in such a way as to serve his individual needs. Assigning the locus of control to within yourself positions you as an architect of your own future. While we cannot control many external factors, we are absolutely in control of how we choose to respond to those factors. All decisions have consequences. The decision maker must accept responsibility for those consequences.

A number of factors contribute to the de-professionalization of medicine. I identify economic pressures, progressive subspecialization, and Generation X's emphasis on balanced life as significant contributors. The growing preference for shift work further commoditizes the physician. In addition, there is a progressively increasing emphasis on technology and science and a progressively decreasing emphasis on relationships and art in the practice of medicine. Put another way, curing is displacing healing as the physician's primary role. Medical training increasingly emphasizes science, technology, computerization, and doing, while placing progressively less emphasis on relationships. The economics of healthcare reinforce this. Building relationships takes time and is under-reimbursed, or not reimbursed, while procedures may be significantly over-reimbursed. Also, the number of medical students choosing primary care as their specialty area of choice is continually decreasing (Biola et al. 2003). With the decline in the emphasis on training primary care physicians, there has evolved a progressive emphasis on science and technology.

Curing versus healing, and science versus art, are two polarities that need to be managed. Currently, I believe they are out of balance. Reimbursement, societal attitudes, and an emphasis on time management all contribute to a significant imbalance in this relationship. It is my personal view that technical competency, no matter how expertly applied, in the absence of human context is singularly without joy. Similarly, the assumed importance of money as a dominant motivating factor is significant. Joy is a derivative of finding meaning and purpose in work. When money becomes the primary objective, joy is significantly diminished. Happiness is a derivative of working to intrinsic motivation. Rewards fail miserably in efforts to induce lasting change. They actually undermine the intrinsic motivation that promotes optimal performance (Malone 1983).

When meaning and purpose are primary, money becomes a derivative benefit. You get in proportion to what you give. As Winston Churchill has been quoted as saying, "You make a living from what you get; you make a life from what you give." Money motivates once, and then it becomes an entitlement. I do not believe that anyone who is reading this book works for money. You can recruit to money, but you do not retain to money.

I believe that most physicians elected to pursue a career in medicine because they wanted to help people. As a derivative of the acculturation process that accompanies physician training, together with the ever-increasing cost of medical education and the influence of economic pressures, this primary motive becomes suppressed as science and technology come to the fore. In essence, physicians are electing to mortgage the doctor-patient relationship in deference to a doctor-disease or a doctor-technology relationship. More important, when what you do is disconnected from what you value, you begin to feel anger, fear, helplessness, and a lack of energy (Quinn 1996). In effect, you become depressed. Many members of the physician community are depressed (Steiger 2006). I believe it is because they are disconnected from their primary sense of purpose. In addition, if an individual's need for intangible remuneration that attends a career of service is not being met, then you had better pay him a lot of money, because why else should he continue to show up for work?

It is critically important to openly discuss the following statement: "It's only about the money…. It's never about the money." I believe that it is never about money. If you engage physicians in a discussion wherein you ask them to tell you about their most recent peak professional experience, the story will invariably be in reference to how they were appreciated, valued, or in some way seen to have made a significant difference. It is never about the day that the check from Blue Cross arrived in the mail. When you are connected to your work, when your work is the expression of your unique contribution, you not only reap the intangible benefits that accrue, but you also find that money shows up at the front door.

There is a need to reestablish this connection between vocational calling and work. To remain disconnected is to choose slow death. There is no other alternative (Quinn 1996).

Malone (1983) wrote the single best book on leadership that I have ever read: *Small Unit Leadership*. In his book, Malone emphasizes the importance of skill, will, and teamwork. He defines "will" as the alignment of self-interest with group interest. "Teamwork" is built on trust. Trust rests on practiced skill and a sense of competence and confidence. Building teamwork aligns group interest with self-interest—that is, doing well together something that matters to the individual. This is very close to Fred Lee's definition of joy: "Working really hard with people you like doing something that matters for somebody else" (2006). Malone further notes that it is productivity that drives morale rather than morale driving productivity. The point he makes is that leadership demands paying attention to and managing the intangibles. When this is done, tangible rewards become a predictable derivative benefit.

I would like to cite two business books in support of my position. These books are arguably two of the most influential books written in the past 15 years. The first book, *Built to Last* (Collins and Porras 1997), applied an academic approach to identifying elements that were held in common by businesses able to sustain a presence in the *Fortune* 500 for greater than 50 years. The authors' conclusion was that, for each of these businesses, the business model only serves as a vehicle for the expression of the core ideology of the workforce. Core ideology was defined as the sum of the organizational vision and values. The other book is titled *Good to Great* (Collins 2001). In this book, a similar academic approach was applied in trying to distinguish characteristics of organizations that outperform well-performing companies in the same business by a ratio of 3:1 using strict economic criteria. The author states that answering the *who* question may be the most important element of performance excellence. This conclusion can be summarized by the metaphor of putting the right people on the bus, letting the wrong people off the bus, seating the right people in the right seats, and then letting them decide where the bus is going to go. In essence, excellence of performance and sustainability are both derivatives of successfully managing intangibles.

As working adults, we spend more time with coworkers than we do with members of our own family. It has never made sense to me why we would not choose to maximize the work environment. I have come to refer to this as "creating sacred places of healing." This originally grew out of an appreciation for the effect of the environment on patient recovery. I have observed that the environment meaningfully affects the quality and the quantity of work performed. I think it is important for individuals to define for their workspace exactly what they stand for and what they will not stand for and to create sacred places of healing in their work environment. This applies equally to the business office or cafeteria as to patient care areas. The process is analogous to the feelings and behaviors evoked when walking into a cathedral or onto a university campus. What are the feelings and behaviors evoked by the expectations defined and modeled in your work area? If the workplace were a sacred place of healing, the healthcare workplace would indeed be joyous.

In an analogous fashion, I would like to distinguish the difference that attends perceiving another person as either a "thou" or a "you." I think it is difficult to behave disrespectfully toward a "thou." It is all too easy to express displeasure toward a "you." Seeing others as "thou" embodies the notion of sacred encounters.

How does this relate to the rapidly changing world of healthcare organization–physician relationships? I believe that these relationships begin with dialogue that allows for the possibility of enhanced mutual understanding and trust. You must explicitly state the purpose of the relationship and the compelling rationale. Identify what you want to create and why. This establishes the vision that is necessary for the creative tension that will propel the initiative forward. Then, the values hierarchy must be defined. What are the principles that will guide decision making going forward? What do you collectively stand for and what will you not stand for? You must identify the metrics that will be used to define progress and success. The clarity of values and metrics will allow individuals to determine if there is a good match between what they care about and what the organization is committed to achieving. It helps guide recruitment and promotes retention, establishes expectations and allows for the application of accountabilities. It defines the *who* of the organization. When these elements are clarified, create the *how* of structure and process. Form must serve function and not inhibit it. The intangibles nourish and sustain relationships and give meaning and purpose to work.

I would like to finish by relating a story that Bill Cosby has told in various instances. When Cosby was attending university, he returned home and sat at the kitchen table with his grandmother. She inquired as to what he had done in class that day. He responded that in philosophy class they had spent three hours discussing the issue of whether the glass is half-full or half-empty. His grandmother responded that it all depends on whether you are drinking or pouring. I think for all of us in healthcare, we need to both individually and on behalf of our organizations answer that very same question about whether we approach the challenges confronting the healthcare industry through a perspective of drinking or pouring.

NOTE

1. QuoteDB, accessed online June 1, 2008, www.quotedb.com/quotes/4152.

REFERENCES

Biola, H., L. A. Green, R. L. Phillips, J. Guirguis-Blake, and G. E. Fryer. 2003. "The U.S. Primary Care Physician Workforce: Persistently Declining Interest in Primary Care Medical Specialties." *American Family Physician* 68: 1484 [Online article; retrieved 6/1/08.] www.graham-center.org/x468.xml

Collins, J. 2001. *Good to Great: Why Some Companies Make the Leap...and Others Don't*. New York: HarperCollins.

Collins, J., and J. Porras. 1997. *Built to Last: Successful Habits of Visionary Companies*. New York: Harper Collins.

Lee, F. 2006. Personal communication with the author.

Malone, D. 1983. *Small Unit Leadership*. Novato, CA: Presidio Press.

Quinn, R. 1996. *Deep Change*. San Francisco: Jossey Bass.

Steiger, W. 2006. "Discouraged Doctors: Doctors Say Morale Is Hurting." *The Physician Executive* November–December.

Terrell, G. 2007. "Can't Get No (Physician) Satisfaction." *The Physician Executive* September–October.

About the Author

Joseph S. Bujak, MD, FACP, currently serves as vice president of medical affairs for Kootenai Medical Center, Coeur d'Alene, Idaho, where he has organizational responsibility for performance improvement and outcomes measurement. He is a frequently requested speaker, facilitator, and consultant on issues related to healthcare organization–physician relationships, physician leadership development, patient safety and clinical quality improvement, and leading and managing transformational change. He and Tom Atchison coauthored the book, *Leading Transformational Change: The Physician-Executive Partnership* (Health Administration Press 2001), and he has published numerous articles on physician culture and behavior. Bujak's past experiences in clinical research, medical education, primary and specialty medical practice, and administration give him a unique breadth of perspective and help establish credibility with the many constituencies within the provider community.